Praise for th

"Pure inspiration."

Shape Magazine

"…provides answers to practically anyone wondering 'What now?' …this worthy collection succeeds very well."

Publishers Weekly

"Hearing others' stories is the most substantial aspect of any support group… It's the universality of the emotions that links these essays and puts the human face on what can be a very scary disease. For all patient health collections."

Library Journal

Other Books by The Healing Project

Voices of Alzheimer's
Voices of Lung Cancer
Voices of Breast Cancer

Voices of Alcoholism

The Healing Companion:
Stories for Courage,
Comfort and Strength

Edited by
The Healing Project
www.thehealingproject.org

"Voices Of" Series Book No. 4

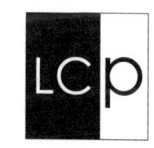

LaChancepublishing

LACHANCE PUBLISHING • NEW YORK
www.lachancepublishing.com

Copyright © 2008 by LaChance Publishing LLC

ISBN 978-1-934184-04-2

Victor Starsia
Managing Editor

Richard Day Gore
Editor

All rights reserved. Printed in the United States of America.

No portion of this book may be reproduced—mechanically, electronically, or by any other means, including photocopying—without the express written permission of the publisher.

Library of Congress Control Number: 2007938288

Publisher: LaChance Publishing LLC
120 Bond Street
Brooklyn, NY 11210
www.lachancepublishing.com

Distributor: Independent Publishers Group
814 North Franklin Street
Chicago, IL 60610
www.ipgbook.com

Ruth Fishel, excerpts from "My Dark Nights of the Soul" from *Living Light as a Feather: How to Find Joy in Every Day and a Purpose in Every Problem*. Copyright © 2004 by Ruth Fishel. Reprinted with the permission of the author and Health Communications, Inc. www.hcibooks.com

All things have a beginning, although the journey from beginning to end is not always clear and straightforward. While work on *Voices Of* began just a short time ago, the seeds were planted long ago by beloved sources. This book is dedicated to Jennie, Larry and Denise, who in the face of all things good and bad gave courage and support in excess. But especially to Richard, who taught us by the way he lived his life that anything is possible given enough time, hard work and love.

Contents

Foreword
    Charles Beem xi

Foreword: *High Society*
    Joseph A. Califano, Jr. xiii

Introduction: *The Healing Project*
    Debra LaChance, Founder xix

Acknowledgments xxv

Part I: FIRST TASTE

As If It Happened Yesterday
    T. Lloyd Reilly 3

The Promise of Hope
    Clay A. Adams 5

Understanding Alcoholism
    Dennis C. Daley, Ph.D. and Antoine Douaihy, M.D. 10

Generations
    Richard Day Gore 11

Sober, Not Dry
    Diane Mierzwick 17

Part II: POWERLESS

Daddy Hyde
    Donna Veneto 23

King Alcohol and His Loyal Subject
  Tracy Alverson 29

A Parent's Trial
  Anne Pascale 35

A Sister's Regret
  Gloria Raskin 41

Two Mothers
  Lisa Dordal 45

The Healing Power of Truth
  Karen W. Waggoner 51

Part III: FAMILY

May Day
  Martha Deborah Hall 59

He's Not an Alcoholic
  Mridu Khullar 61

The Whites of His Eyes
  Leslie Smith Townsend 65

Family Tree
  Katrina Cleveland 75

I Really Am Special
  Julie Anne Hunter 81

Mothers Can't Be Drunks, Can They?
  Valerie Scully 87

The Day He Left
  Allison S. Jones 95

Guilty Feet Have Got No Rhythm
  Angela Lovell 99

Part IV: I NEED HELP

The Path Was Rocky (But Worth It)
Steven Michael Sarber 109

Amazing Grace
Dagan Elizabeth Manahl 113

Losing Control
Jessica Saldivar 119

To Drink or Not To Drink
Lisa Schoonover 123

Buzz
Miriam Lee 129

My Story
Yvette Fitzjarrald 135

My Demon
Mary C. White 141

Part V: LEARNING TO LIVE

The Wake Up Call
Sheri Ables 147

No Longer in Charge
Christine Valentine 153

A Mother's Journal
Susan Norton 157

Reason to Believe
Ginger B. Collins 165

Breaking Point
Tiffany Williams 173

The Journey to Hope
Uma Girish 179

Part VI: MIRACLE

Do You Know the Way to A.A.?
Diane Saarinen 187

My Dark Nights of the Soul
Ruth Fishel 189

A Simple Cup of Coffee
Lucy Brummett 195

Reprieve from Insanity
Peter Wright 199

Desperation
Kim Mallin 207

Do As I Say, Not As I Do
Ed Lamp, Ph.D. 213

Blessed by Truth
Hannah Smith 217

Till Death Do We Part
Katrina Hunt 223

Better than Better
Leslie C. Lewis 229

Drunk
Sara Ekks 235

A Look to the Future of Alcoholism Treatment
Ron L. Alterman, M.D. 243

Afterword: *Caregiver, Heal Thyself*
James Huysman, Psy.D. 249

Resources 257

Foreword
Charles Beem

A man on a business trip in Ohio was experiencing the desperate craving of alcohol withdrawal and wasn't sure what to do. He knew he needed to talk to another alcoholic, but didn't know anyone in that unfamiliar town. Finally, an arrangement was made for him to meet a physician who also had a significant drinking problem. As a way of introduction, Bill Wilson told Dr. Bob Smith his story. Something magical happened. It wasn't just a person telling his story to an uninterested party. There was listening. The events of one person's story became a metaphor for the other. There was true sharing. A synergy happened. The truth of their individual stories transcended the names, places, and dates, and became a vehicle for survival for them and, eventually, millions of people throughout the world.

The ancient tradition of telling one's story in a fellowship creates a truth, a wholeness, a sense of knowing, that goes beyond dates, times, and events. Richard J. Caron, founder of Caron Treatment Services, knew that truth and told it not only face-to-face, but in the form of his free newsletter—*Chit Chat*. Eventually, he raised enough funds to start a treatment program that has grown to a place that exceeded his wildest dreams. It becomes the essence of survival for those who participate.

What are your dreams? Tell your story and really hear the stories of others. Be guided by spiritual principles. Be open to your own truth as well as your own falsehoods.

If you choose to read this book, look beyond the names, dates, places, and plot lines. Look, instead, into the truth of the stories. You might find your survival and, eventually, your dreams.

Charles Beem is the Executive Director of Adult Services of Caron, a nationally recognized not-for-profit chemical dependency treatment organization located in Wernersville, Pennsylvania. He directs all aspects of adult treatment services at Caron.

Foreword
High Society
Joseph A. Califano, Jr.

On any given day, 100 million Americans are self-medicating with alcohol or illegal substances like marijuana, cocaine, heroin, methamphetamines, hallucinogens, Ecstasy and other designer drugs, inhaling from aerosol cans or glue bottles, smoking or taking some stimulant, antidepressant, tranquillizer or painkiller. The abuse of and addiction to mind-altering drugs is America's public health enemy number one. Alcohol abuse and addiction alone claim 16 to 20 million people. Some 100,000 Americans die each year from alcoholism and alcohol abuse; 470,000 die from tobacco and other drug abuse. The mortality and morbidity toll and personal tragedies from addictive disorders would be regarded as a pandemic if any other illness were involved. Yet, in the U.S. today, alcohol or other drug addiction is more likely to be ignored, misunderstood, stigmatized or punished than effectively treated.

Addiction is a chronic disease with physical, psychological, emotional and spiritual elements that require continuing and holistic care. It is a disease of the brain that dramatically affects behavior, and a chronic disease more like diabetes and high blood pressure than like a broken arm or influenza. It cannot be fixed or cured in a single round of therapy, with a surgical procedure or one regimen of pharmaceuticals.

But, there is good news. As with diabetes or hypertension, people suffering from addiction can and do learn to manage their illness and live healthy, productive lives. Long-term disease management is as critical to treating the alcoholic or other drug addict as are lifestyle changes and taking insulin or hypertensive pills to managing diabetes or hypertension.

Our failure to recognize that addiction can be prevented and effectively treated costs our nation close to one trillion dollars per year in health care, low productivity, disability, welfare, fires, crime and punishment, property damage from vandalism, interest on the federal debt, legal and court costs, family break-up, child abuse, and the array of social interventions, public and private, to deal with the ravages of this epidemic. The human misery that addiction and abuse cause can't be calculated—the broken homes, teen mothers and absent fathers, the young and old alike victimized by violence, lost opportunities and lives prematurely snuffed out.

While the stories in this book are about alcoholism, the underlying issue is addiction, regardless of the substance of abuse. There is a statistical and biological (chemical, neurological) relationship between abusing alcohol, smoking, and marijuana use, and between abuse of these drugs and use of cocaine, heroin, controlled prescription drugs, methamphetamines, hallucinogens and other substances. Those who are addicted to alcohol or abuse it regularly are far likelier to smoke and abuse other drugs than people who are not alcohol abusers or addicts. For example, 9th through 12th graders who report drinking and smoking at least once in the last month are 30 times more likely to smoke marijuana than those who did not drink or smoke, and those who drank, smoked cigarettes and used marijuana at least once in the past month were more than 17 times more likely to use another drug like cocaine, heroin or LSD.

Research has shown that all drugs of abuse affect similar pathways in the brain, increasing dopamine and producing feelings of pleasure. And, for many teens in particular, drinking, smoking and other drug use often is a symptom of incipient depression, anxiety or some other (usually undiagnosed) mental illness that hikes the risk of drug abuse. So when we think about treating an alcohol problem, it is critical to address the misuse of other drugs and the mental health issues that may influence the chances of recovery.

Substance abuse and addiction lurk just beyond the welcome mat in many homes. Alcohol is implicated in most instances of domestic violence. Even a non-violent alcohol- or other drug-abusing family member sends shock waves into every corner of the house. Children are innocent victims of untreated parental substance abuse. The damage begins in the womb of mothers who drink, smoke and use other drugs during pregnancy. Fetal alcohol syndrome is among the top three causes of the birth defects associated with mental retardation.

Untreated addiction increases the risk of child neglect and abuse, and children growing up in homes where addiction is present are likelier to end up in foster care, turn to alcohol and other drugs themselves, and land in the juvenile justice system. And, substance abuse is too often a ticket to jail or prison. Most violent crimes—murders, assaults, vehicular homicides, child molestations and rapes—are prompted, abetted or aggravated by alcohol and other drugs. Alcohol abuse is the most wanted criminal. Addiction haunts the welfare rolls, pummels public housing and is a constant companion of the homeless, and it is implicated in the five leading causes of death in America today. Our failure to understand the pervasive culpability of substance abuse and addiction to these social problems has led to public policies that shovel up the consequences rather than prevent or treat the cause.

Unfortunately, treatment services in this country are relatively scarce and often ineffective. Less than 17% of those in need of addiction treatment receive any type of services and there is no way to assure the quality of services they do receive.

There are steps we can and should take to address this enormous public health problem. One major step is to keep young people from starting to drink and abuse alcohol or use other drugs. The overwhelming majority of alcoholics and other drug abusers in the U.S. today began using before they reached the age of 21. A child who gets through age 21 without abusing alcohol or prescription drugs, using illegal drugs or smoking is virtually certain never to do so. All drug pushers, be they alcohol or tobacco industry executives or illegal street or Internet dealers, understand this. They've known for decades how important it is to persuade kids to try their stuff. The tragedy is that so many politicians, public health professionals and parents either don't get it or don't act on it.

We need a fundamental change in attitude among all people—parents, politicians and professionals—about substance abuse and addiction. We must end our denial, stamp out the stigma, reshape our medical system, rethink our concepts of crime and punishment, and commit the energy and resources needed to confront this disease. Failure to do so is a decision to write off millions of Americans and continue imposing on taxpayers exorbitant medical, social service and prison costs.

The task of preventing teen substance abuse is largely a Mom-and-Pop operation. Parent power is the most potent, the least appreciated, and the most underutilized resource we have in the struggle to raise children free of alcohol and other drug abuse. The front line of America's addiction problem is not in legislative hearing rooms or courtrooms run by politicians and judges. It is in living rooms and dining rooms, and across kitchen tables, in the hands of parents and families.

The medical and public health professionals have done an abysmal job in educating the American people about the medical reality of alcohol and other drug addiction. Their failure to instruct the nation about addiction as they have about AIDS permits us to treat those afflicted with this disease as the biblical lepers of modern-day America. There are two sure-fire ways to effect the basic cultural change needed to get the medical profession to accord substance abuse and addiction the appropriate attention as a chronic disease. One is to recognize as malpractice the failure of physicians to screen for the disease and diagnose it and, upon such a diagnosis, the failure to treat the patient or refer the patient for treatment. The other is to require health insurers to cover treatment costs and reimburse physicians for time spent talking to patients.

The faith community has an important role to play since the combination of science-based treatment and spiritual practice produces more hope and better results for millions struggling with this disease. Political leadership also is essential and it is time to abandon the cautious, step-by-step approach and take some giant leaps.

We need to change public policy to be sure that people coming into our health care, welfare, child welfare, juvenile and criminal justice and other social service systems are screened and assessed for substance abuse and addiction and co-occurring mental health problems, and get effective treatment. There are many promising practices such as screenings and brief interventions, drug courts, age and gender specific treatments and family therapies that can be employed.

We also need to create a strong profession to assure and continually improve quality services. The field of substance abuse and addiction treatment has never been subjected to the demanding standards of professional preparation for entry and continuing practice that characterize the medical profession: extensive graduate education with academic and clinical components, tough licensing exams, continuing-education requirements, and oversight by professional boards in each state. Many methods of treatment for substance abuse have never been systematically subjected to the kind of peer-reviewed, scientifically based outcome research that has produced high quality in medical and surgical procedures.

What we need today is a dramatic shift in our nation's attitude toward alcohol and other drug abuse and addiction. This is the subject of my latest book, *High Society: How Substance Abuse Ravages America and What to Do About It*. This book calls for a revolution in the way all of us—parents and physicians, teens, schools and universities, clergy, cops and corporations, judges, lawyers, policymakers and journalists—perceive the threat that substance abuse and addiction pose to our people and the obligation to protect our children. It is a call to sober up the High Society, to accept addiction as a chronic disease and recognize its impact on the most intractable domestic problems we confront. It is a call to reform our health care, criminal justice and social service systems; to make the kind of major investment in substance abuse research that we have made in cancer, cardiovascular disease and AIDS; and to reclaim families. By responding to this call, we can improve the quality of life of our people and by example of others across the world.

Joseph A. Califano, Jr. is Chairman and President of The National Center on Addiction and Substance Abuse (CASA) at Columbia University, and former Secretary of the U.S. Department of Health, Education and Welfare. He is the author of *High Society: How Substance Abuse Ravages America and What to Do About It*, recently released by PublicAffairs™, a member of the Perseus Books Group and available through Amazon.com, Barnes & Noble, and www.casacolumbia.org. All royalties from sales of the book are donated to CASA at Columbia University.

Introduction
The Healing Project
Debra LaChance

I wanted to ask the people around me, "Would you please raise your hand if you feel as isolated as I do?" Walking the busy streets of Manhattan on a beautiful sunny day, I was surrounded by people but I'd never felt so alone. Just minutes before, my doctors had broken the news to me that I had a particularly aggressive form of breast cancer.

Since moving to New York from a small town in Rhode Island, I'd had my share of ups and downs but had always risen to the challenges that living and working in New York can bring. But on this summer afternoon, I felt as if the world was suddenly rushing past me while I seemed to be moving in slow motion; I was completely alone.

After recovering from the initial shock I found that one of the first things I almost automatically began to look for, besides doctors, was a sense of connection. I needed to hear from other people who had gone through what I was experiencing, who truly understood what it meant and who might be able to help. I wasn't ready for a regular support group, and with surgery and treatment looming, I simply didn't have the time. But I am an avid reader, and I assumed that finding the personal stories of those who had gone through this ordeal before me would be relatively easy. But there seemed to be a vacuum; almost nothing. Where were the *real people* to talk to? Where was the literature that wasn't just about the hardcore science of the disease, but about how to cope?

There was one book that gave me great solace, *Just Get Me Through This* by Deborah Cohen and Robert A. Gelfand. It was more of a personal story, rather than a clinical one, and it created in me a desire for more stories that get to the heart of the emotional experience, that help the reader through it. I knew there must be countless others out there who needed to tell their stories—and to hear the stories of others as well. I decided that part of my own, ongoing healing process would be to find a way to bring people like me together, to create some kind of forum where these real stories could be shared.

Over time my vision of community crystallized and *The Healing Project* was born. I'd already realized that having access to the real stories of real people would make the journey through breast cancer much easier to endure. My thoughts kept returning to that walk through Manhattan after I'd heard my diagnosis and that feeling of terrible loneliness. As sympathetic as friends and loved ones could be, I felt that no one could truly understand this journey except someone who had made it before. I was convinced that getting and giving courage, comfort, and strength were as important as good medical care, and I became determined to help build a community for people like me who were undergoing the terribly isolating experience of dealing with a life-threatening or chronic disease. This would be *The Healing Project*'s mission: to become a bridge across which people can make those all-important emotional connections.

And those are the people I want to help me build *The Healing Project* community. I began to develop *The Healing Project* as a place where people can contribute funds for research, time for connecting with others, and most of all, a place to share their stories. Since then, *The Healing Project* has been collecting stories by those touched by illness or diseases for books like this one: books that inspire and inform for the road ahead and impart a sense of community for those caught up in dealing with the moment. When you're sick or afraid, it's a godsend to know that there are others who understand. These books are meant to be a companion for patients, their friends, and families, an oasis where they can find strength in shared experiences.

In addition to the books, we're also working on other initiatives through *The Healing Project*, including Voices Who Care, a "virtual support group" which will allow family and friends to connect with others in real time. I don't want anyone to have to feel the way I did the day of my diagnosis when I was walking through the city alone and afraid. There's so much strength in others—you just have to find them.

When you are dealing with disease, you have to be ready to chart a new course, for the rest of your life, no matter what the outcome. And it helps to see that others are busy charting their own courses along with you. That's what these stories are all about. Reading these amazing contributions to the *Voices Of* series convinces me that I don't really have a uniquely remarkable story at all.

The truth is *everyone* does.

Debra LaChance is the creator and founder of *The Healing Project*.

The Healing Project

Individuals diagnosed with life-threatening or chronic, debilitating illness face countless physical, emotional, social, spiritual, and financial challenges during their treatment and throughout their lives. The support of family members, friends, and the community at large is essential to their successful recovery and their quality of life; access to accurate and current information about their illnesses enables patients and their caregivers to make informed decisions about treatment and post-treatment care. Founded in 2005 by Debra LaChance, *The Healing Project* is dedicated to promoting the health and well-being of these individuals, developing resources to enhance their quality of life, and supporting the family members and friends who care for them. *The Healing Project* creates ways in which individuals can share their stories while providing access to current information about their illnesses, and strives to promote public understanding of the impact such illnesses have on the lives of those affected. For more information about *The Healing Project* and its programs, please visit our website at www.thehealingproject.org.

Acknowledgments

This book would not have been possible without the selfless dedication of many people giving freely of their valuable time and expertise. We'd particularly like to thank Theresa Russell, Alice Bergmann and Amy Shore for their unending efforts to reach out to the people and organizations making so many contributions to this book; Melissa Marr for her invaluable assistance, insights and opinions; and to Drs. Dennis C. Daley, Antoine Douaihy and Ron L. Alterman for lending their extraordinary expertise; and to the many, many people who submitted their stories to us, for their courage, their generosity and their humanity.

Part I

My grandfather handed a drink to my sister for a sip...
I recall a feeling of delight that seemed to speak to me...
my very *first taste* *of alcohol...*

As If It Happened Yesterday
T. Lloyd Reilly

Many tell me they think it is impossible to remember something that long ago; I had to have been too young. I had not even started to talk. How could I possibly remember the first time I got drunk?

Well, I do. My family and I were at my grandfather's house in New Jersey. It was spring or summer. My sister and I were sitting on the picnic table in the backyard. My grandfather handed a beer to my sister for a "sip." At the time, for the northeastern Irish-Catholic, it seemed that drinking was not as dangerous as it is known to be today. A man came home from work and drank a beer to wash down the effects of the day: dust from the road, sweat from his labor, frustration at not making enough money. With an absent father, we children yearned for the company of the men in our family; my grandfather and my favorite uncle were the male influences in our young lives. They drank, and we wanted to be just like them, the men that held us, hugged us, and told us we were beautiful and worthy.

As the afternoon went on, we asked for more "sips" of the beer in Poppy's hand. My sister, who held me in her arms, put me down whenever she was delivered the dark amber bottle. I reached for the bottle and we struggled for a minute. Poppy scolded my sister and told her to give it to me. I tilted the bottle to my lips and drank deeply (I never have understood the concept of a "sip"—how someone could just take a little when he could have a lot). The taste of this infusion of malt and hops captured me, held me in its grip, and has never left me. I recall a feeling of delight that seemed to speak to me, telling me that nothing mattered or would ever matter, as long as I kept drinking; I remember Poppy scolding me for emptying the bottle. All I wanted at the time was to inhabit the place that the beer took me. All there was at that moment, and for the next forty years, was euphoria. Ecstasy in a bottle, which could be found in every refrigerator of every house in which I ever lived.

Strange as it may sound, I thought of that day every time I popped a tab, mixed a drink, or tipped a bottle to my lips. I never understood why the memory of that day was held with so much intensity within me. A few years ago, about the time of the tenth anniversary of the miracle of my recovery, I discovered the answer. At a family birthday and barbecue, we sat around the table after eating, telling stories of the family. This evolved into home movie viewing and browsing the family photo albums. In one album I came upon a picture of that very day. I looked at my sister, and felt remorse for the pain of her tears. I looked at my dear grandfather smiling, and I stared at myself holding the bottle to my lips. The year the picture was taken was written underneath. The date astonished me: 1954. I thought of all those times I brought that bottle to my mouth. I thought of all the times I woke to the overwhelming need to get to that next "sip" in spite of the illness it caused. I thought of a young child who just wanted to feel better, and did not know why. And I thought of my birthday: June 21, 1953.

T. Lloyd Reilly is a writer and schoolteacher who has been an alcoholic and addict all of his life. Eleven years in recovery, he actively participates in a twelve-step program, gratefully offering his experience, strength and hope to all who would seek a better life.

The Promise of Hope
Clay A. Adams

The van skidded to a stop, digging into the mud on the rain-soaked roadside. Despite the jolt from the vehicle's brakes, I remained asleep. With a roar the van door slid open, rupturing my slumber. Gathering my senses and my gear, I made my way past the front seats and reluctantly stepped onto Interstate 45 southbound in Houston, Texas.

A frozen rain battered my face. With a makeshift spear in one hand and a trash bag in the other, I took the first step of the four-mile trek ahead of me. I harpooned an empty beer can that floated in a nearby puddle. How fitting, I thought to myself. But I was coming to realize that walking four miles down the interstate in the freezing rain to clean up litter was the best place for me to be at six o'clock on a Friday morning.

The word "average" describes my adolescence well. You certainly wouldn't expect to find me in any so-called "at-risk" group. But it didn't matter who I was—my struggles erupted out of who I feared I wasn't. I had three older brothers. Two were more on the wild side. It was they who invited me to experience my very first taste of alcohol. As their younger brother I had forever endured their teasing, rejection, ridicule and abuse. This could break that cycle; I would be one of them! Once I had resigned myself to thinking that way, the liquor didn't sting so much. You acquire the taste after three or four and it's downhill from there.

The effect of diving into that bottle was profound. Fear and worry disappeared, cares went far away, ordinary events became exciting, boring situations turned hilarious. Not only would alcohol's magical properties keep me coming back for more, they overpowered even the strongest sense of guilt.

Before long, I had established a comfortable routine that would invariably place me at my brothers' apartment. Because I still lived at home with my parents, it was often necessary to lie and manipulate my way around various house rules that might prevent me from being available to drink. First I was drinking once or twice every couple of weeks. By that summer, I was drinking and partying with my brothers almost every day.

Soon, I was living life to the fullest and loving every minute of it. Just when I thought I had found nirvana, my brothers introduced me to yet another new mind-altering substance. After some deliberation, they placed in my hand a small marble pipe with a freshly packed bowl of marijuana. After a very short period of reluctance and uneasiness, I decided to try it. The drug obliterated my inhibitions. Apathy took hold. I delved deeper and deeper into the realm of this newfound high.

I spent the rest of my summer vacation indulging in my vices. My final two years in high school marked a rapid and steady decline. My grades fell sharply and my teachers grew concerned about my well being. I ended up in trouble at school and, more frequently, with my parents. I cared less and less for outside activities that might reduce my precious partying time. Alcohol became more important than my studies, my family and even most of my friends.

The following summer, I fully crossed the bridge from using alcohol to abusing it. I was accepted into a good university, paid for by my parents. For me, college wasn't just an opportunity to better myself and bolster my future business ventures. It was my first taste of true freedom. I could drink to my heart's content.

I also discovered several new drugs while in college. My lifestyle was shared by a host of fellow students, many of whom would later form my new circle of friends. We ventured off to the keg parties on the weekends, spent weeknights out at discreet locations smoking pot and drinking malt liquor.

I decided drinking was much more personally rewarding than attending class; my grade point average dropped to an abysmal low. When I ran out of money, I sold my books to buy more booze. Drugs weren't cheap either, so I needed a financial solution to support that habit as well. I discovered that my student loan was not entirely used up by tuition that year. I blew almost all of it on liquor and beer, making sure to set aside a little for the coming weeks. Once that money was gone, I used my credit card to buy books, turning right around and selling them for cash. Soon I was selling pot on campus, which drew the attention of law enforcement and a drug task force. A few months later the task force had me in custody for minor offenses and I spent a week in jail.

My final semester was miserable. I lived off campus in an apartment with a drinking buddy. When we went to bed, we would set up the bottle and shot glasses for the next morning so we could get an early start drinking before class. Not surprisingly, I failed all my classes, again. All of my time, money and resources had gone to support my alcoholism. I violated the terms of my academic probation for a third time, spent more time in jail and remained under police surveillance.

Consequence had caught up with me. I returned home filled with shame and self-pity. Not long afterwards, I reunited with my old drinking friends and spent a good deal of time out partying. One day, my parents confronted me about my so-called problem. I denied it. Nevertheless, my mother kicked me out of the house and vowed I could only return on the condition that I go into rehab. Faced with the choice between the street and a treatment center, I chose the street.

An old friend took pity on me and let me stay in his apartment. But eventually he got fed up with my ways and he left for Austin. At the end of that month I was evicted. I spent two nights utterly homeless. But I had plenty of liquor, a six pack of beer and a pinch of marijuana. So I drove with my last remaining friend to a quiet spot along the banks of a bayou. I had hit many bottoms on the way down, but this time I had truly arrived. There I sat, angry, defeated, groggy, dazed, saturated with toxins and far from sane. I told my friend I was going home. I was sick and tired of being sick and tired. I popped open a beer and clasped one more joint between my lips. I glanced solemnly at my friend, swearing to a conviction I'd uttered so many times in vain. "This is my last joint, and my last beer... ever."

When our session ended, I threw the bottle in the woods and flicked the joint into the creek below. Then I broke down in tears. A short while later, I took the longest walk of my life: up the pathway to my parent's home. I lifted a trembling fist to the door and knocked softly, almost wishing no one would answer. Moments later, I was reunited with my family after a long tour of unspeakable suffering. My mother steadfastly upheld her vow. She allowed me to spend that night in the house with the assurance that I would be taken to a treatment center first thing in the morning. Broken, beaten and out of options, I accepted.

The next morning my father woke me up at 8 o'clock and rushed me to dress and pack some clothing. By 8:30 we were heading for the Texas House, a drug and alcohol rehabilitation center in northwest Houston. It seemed like something that I could handle, until we arrived. Life was hard enough with a head full of booze. Coping with life in sobriety was unimaginable to me. Nevertheless, I somehow composed myself and accompanied my father into the Clinical Supervisor's office. He questioned me about my lifestyle and behavior. Once he'd concluded his interview, I was told I would be accepted if I chose to reside there and follow the rules. The counselor asked me if I had any questions that might help me decide. I only had one: "What should I expect to get out of living here in treatment?" Without hesitation, the counselor spoke firmly and compassionately with a single sentence I will never forget.

"You will comprehend the word *serenity* and you will know peace."

Picking up trash on the side of the road would become my daily occupation for eight months. This was my payment for residence at Texas House and a testament to my willingness to strive toward sobriety no matter what the condition. For the first time, I had done something different. I had made a sacrifice. I paid a short-term price for a long-term reward. I removed chemicals from my life and replaced them with a God of my understanding.

Today, I have clarity. I have peace and serenity. I acquired many tangible blessings as well—things like a good job, my own place to live, my own vehicle, a beautiful wife and much, much more. I could never list every gift I've been given as a result of sobriety and God's presence in my life. But I will list one more. That gift is the experience itself. It was promised to me, when I committed to recovery, that there was hope for me. It was promised to me that my experience would some day benefit others. Because you see, it has afforded me a unique opportunity to offer this testimony. So confident am I that a better life awaits us all that I extend to you the same promise of hope. Just remember: Pain may very well be necessary. Suffering is optional.

Born and raised in Houston, Clay A. Adams lives with his wife in Whitehouse, Texas and works as a transportation coordinator for a national corporation. A new writer, the author is also a poet, photographer and chess enthusiast.

Understanding Alcoholism

Dennis C. Daley, Ph.D.
and Antoine Douaihy, M.D.

Alcoholism is a significant public health problem as well as a disease. It is associated with injuries, accidents, a variety of medical problems and premature death, psychiatric disorders such as depression, and social problems such as crime and family breakups. These and other effects of the disease cost society hundreds of billions of dollars per year in lost job productivity and the increased use of social services. As a result, understanding alcoholism, its causes, treatment and the potential for recovery is of paramount importance to addicted individuals, their families, and to society as a whole.

(continued on page 28)

Generations
Richard Day Gore

From an Instant Message conversation with a friend.

JK56: Top o' the evening. How's by you?

RDG: Quiet. How are things going down there?

JK56: Grrr. Liz had to go to Belmar this afternoon to bring Beth back, right in the middle of Senior Week.

RDG: ???????

JK56: She and her friends were evicted from their rental. "Unauthorized guests."

RDG: WTF! Man...

JK56: So there went the $300 we gave her for graduation.

RDG: Who was the Perp?

JK56: Her friends, although I believe there are other unsaid details.

RDG: Aren't there always?

JK56: Yup. I was on the phone with her last night. Outright defiance. She said several times she was not going to leave; after about

30 minutes, I convinced her otherwise and Liz went to bring her home. Not back yet, can't wait, nice way to punctuate a long lousy work day. It's emotionally draining for both of us, especially since we absolutely know there was booze involved.

RDG: Teenagers away for Senior Week? How could there not be?

JK56: Exactly.

RDG: How old is she?

JK56: 17.

RDG: 17, of course!!! God help you, my friend.

JK56: Disappointing. And scary, too. Anyway... hopefully a lesson was learned. But who knows, this ain't exactly *Leave It to Beaver*.

RDG: Sounds more like *24*! Let me know how it works out, Agent Bauer.

JK56: Will do. I hate this stuff; it reminds me of growing up, in the worst ways.

RDG: Your dad?

JK56: Yeah. When alcohol colors your childhood like it did mine, it's hard not to worry all the time when you have kids. I mean come on, you know kids are going to drink if they get the chance, and you can only hope and pray that it doesn't get out of hand.

RDG: But you and Liz set good examples, don't you?

JK56: We try to, but it's worrisome and frankly when an alcohol issue comes up, it's hard not to get steaming mad like I did years ago because of my dad. Whatever, I'm sure I had it better than a lot of kids who had a drunk parent. At least I got most of it out of my system in college. Most of it.

RDG: Yes, I remember. I was actually a bit envious of your partying while I stayed at home like the geek I was.

JK56: Oh yeah, envious of a hangover.

RDG: Well, they don't hurt as much when you're young.

JK56: No. The hurt is what got me drinking in the first place. You know. Family tradition.

RDG: But at least you stayed serious about school.

JK56: Mostly serious. I believe it was because of my precarious economic position.

RDG: How so?

JK56: At that time, being dependent on my father… it was pretty shaky at home. I believed we could be on the street at any moment.

RDG: Man…

JK56: For years. Elementary school, junior high, high school, it just got worse and worse.

RDG: A powerful motivator, for good or bad, depending.

JK56: In my case, both. I was pissed at how Dad's drinking was affecting my mother, pissed that I had to deal with it as a kid… So of course I drank as soon as I got away from the house!

RDG: Funny how that works, except of course it's not funny at all.

JK56: Right. And believe me, with Dad's example and the anger and the pressure, I pretty much thought that you drank specifically to get shitfaced. I'd pop one and just keep downing them until I was wasted. Anyway, the positive thing is that I was smart enough to realize pretty early that I needed vocational training in case I ended up becoming the Responsible Party at home.

RDG: Wow, we knew there was a problem at your place, but back then people didn't talk about it. I can't imagine worrying that the responsibilities of a household with three kids and a mother might crash down on you at any moment. What a way for a kid to live.

JK56: Yeah, unbelievable pressure, relentless. I really did think that my dad was going to just pick up and go, or cave in and be unable to provide. Or die. Suffice it to say, he was a tough guy to be around.

RDG: Violent?

JK56: He could be, but that wasn't it. It was witnessing the degeneration right in front of you and not being able to do anything about it. "Frustrating" just doesn't express it. It was utterly, completely, totally demoralizing. Spiritually depleting.

RDG: For all those years, what an awful experience.

JK56: Maybe I shoulda cleared out after high school, joined the Army or something. But I didn't have the confidence to do that. I didn't think I could do anything for a long time. I had food, shelter, clothing and love from Mom keeping me at home—and like I said, the need to be there to protect her just in case. And to be fair, I did get tough love from Dad. But the sights, sounds (and smells) of alcoholism... and to see that inflicted on your mother. Not good. Sucks the confidence right out of you to see your own father, who's supposed to be the ultimate good example, passed out on the front step in a pool of, well... unpleasantness. Not inside where the neighbors can't see, mind you, but in broad daylight, right where the paperboy leaves the paper, while Mrs. Pierson lurks in her window eager to telegraph the news to one and all.

RDG: I can't imagine.

JK56: Yeah, imagine coming home from school and carrying him in with your little brother while the neighbors watch. Knowing that your mother is going to cry, that the kids at school are going to be talking about it behind your back tomorrow. What does that do to you? How can it not make you angry all the time? And when I say all the time, I mean *all the time.*

RDG: Well you've certainly mellowed out, and we all find your remaining edge quite endearing.

JK56: I can think of a few car windshields that would disagree.

RDG: ?????

JK56: I smashed 3 car windshields out of sheer rage. From the inside. Just like the Incredible Hulk, kicking and punching them out. I'd drink, and it would just blow the lid right off every leftover frustration from my childhood.

RDG: At least you weren't smashing people.

JK56: Nope. And believe me, I know I'm lucky I didn't break any of those windshields with my head at 70 miles per hour.

RDG: Man, I had no idea. What turned you around? I mean, where did the anger go?

JK56: Church and family helped defuse it, but it took a while. Plus I'm an overworked executive and it's an inefficient use of my time and energy. Thank God I never got so wasted that I forgot my responsibilities to others.

RDG: Just like in high school!

JK56: Right. They say alcoholism doesn't ever go away, and my dad's example has definitely been breathing down my neck for what seems like my whole life, keeping my nose on that grindstone. So in a way I haven't had a break in, like, 40 years.

RDG: Good thing you don't deal with pressure the same way you used to.

JK56: Amen. Let me tell you, you walk a tightrope as a parent when it comes to alcohol. I've tried to give my kids a home that has all the stability that mine didn't. But when stuff like this

Belmar thing comes up, the worry wheels definitely go into overdrive. I can't get it out of my mind; it's been weighing on me since Beth entered her teens. You know, the idea that somewhere, at some time, she's going to have that first drink, and not knowing where it's going to lead. Try telling a kid that something's bad for them. If you'd tried talking a beer out of my hand back in college, I'd have told you to stick it.

RDG: Or smashed my windshield.

JK56: Hey, the damned windshields had it coming, okay? Seriously, though, think about it. There I was drinking to escape from the problems my family experienced because of my father's drinking! That's how badly alcohol can screw up your perceptions and your life. Every single day I pray that Beth understands that, but kids seem to prefer to learn the important stuff the hard way. Like I did.

RDG: Well you turned out fine and I'm sure your kids will, too.

JK56: Fingers crossed, toes crossed, knock wood, rabbit's foot in my pocket.

RDG: At least you're not saying "I'll drink to that."

JK56: Point taken. And there's the car. Gotta go.

Richard Day Gore moved from Virginia to Manhattan to pursue a writing career, then took a lengthy detour into the fashion industry. He now writes for advertising agencies and websites, and is the Senior Editor at LaChance Publishing. He counts among his greatest joys the opportunity to read the many remarkable stories that fill the *Voices Of* book series.

Sober, Not Dry
Diane Mierzwick

During high school, my group would get together on Friday nights and cruise the nearby city. After a week of homework and sports, it was nice to be with friends, sing to the radio and laugh about nothing in particular. On one of those nights, our classmate Tim drove us in his souped-up Impala to a local lookout point where, below us, we could see the shimmering city lights. Then another classmate, Charles, pulled a grocery bag from under the front seat and said, "Surprise!"

Charles had stolen several beers from his sister's fridge. He opened each of the three cans and passed them to us in the back seat. My girlfriend Jeanette would not take a drink because we were going back to her house at the end of the evening and her parents always waited up for us. But I did. The beer made my eyes water and I shivered with each swallow, but I was able to choke down half the can. No fireworks exploded in my head. No calming sensations warmed my body. Instead, I ended up worrying that I had consumed all those calories for nothing. We headed home.

Jeanette's father casually wandered from his bedroom door to greet us as we stumbled into the house and down the hall. He asked the obligatory questions: Did we have a good time? Where had we gone? Suddenly, I had an answer for every question. I felt like I could talk to Jeanette's dad for the rest of the evening. Thankfully,

Jeanette maneuvered between us and got me into her room. That's when the giggling started. I had found the elixir to my ailment, to my seemingly lifelong feeling of being out of place, of never having the right thing to say, of being uncomfortable around most people. Suddenly it was gone! And all it had taken was a few cans of beer.

After that night and through the rest of high school, there was little time to drink. Playing sports, being a member of the student council and working a part-time job kept me busy and alcohol-free. But soon after high school, I married a man six years older than I. Suddenly, I was thrust into adulthood and seduced by the myth that alcohol would bring a sophistication to my life that I had not gained from experience.

Since I married young and had no children to tie me to home, Happy Hour always seemed to turn into an all-night affair. On hot summer days, after I spent time working in the yard or riding my bike, a beer always tasted good to me. That first swallow soothed my body with the knowledge that relaxation was on the way. It only took a few more to make me feel elated. Then, suddenly it was late at night and I was feeling sick, or it was the next morning and I was feeling sick.

For years, I would tell my husband that I thought I had a drinking problem. He always tried to reassure me. "I've seen you drink only a few and stop," he would tell me, "You don't have a problem." I asked my friends, who also happened to be my drinking buddies. "You only drink on the weekends," they would say, "We're all letting go a little. There's no harm in that." But over the years, especially on all those mornings after, when my head was pounding or I was too sick to take the dogs for their jog, I could feel my sense of self-respect slowly eroding. So eventually I quit drinking, what they call being "dry" as opposed to really being sober. For two years, I abstained from drinking and enjoyed feeling healthy and being productive.

Then one spring day, with the warm sun shining on my face, I decided that nothing would go better with that feeling of warmth than a cold one. Everyone was happy to see me drinking again. A friend ran to the store in the middle of the day to be sure she had my favorite beer on hand. My husband told me he had missed this side of me. I wondered why I had ever stopped.

But the hangovers and the shame hounded me again. After that day I worked at only having three beers, then drinking water. I paced myself with the lightest drinker in the group. I didn't drink until everyone else had finished one. I didn't drink after ten o'clock. But I always ended up drinking too much.

One summer, I bought a book on alcoholism. I read about people losing their jobs, their families, and about how much they drank, gallons of wine, quarts of vodka. I convinced myself that I wasn't an alcoholic. After all, I hadn't lost anything: I still had my job, I had my husband and my son, and by any standard I lived very well. None of the people in the book were like me. I only drank a few beers, maybe a six pack at the most.

But slowly, alcohol drained away my belief in myself. My health began to suffer. After too many drinks I would have red, blotchy cheeks that lasted three or four days. I was puffy and bloated. I was always exhausted. Just as I was getting over the symptoms of drinking too much, the weekend would arrive, and I would be drinking too much again. When I was not drunk, I was hypersensitive to any perceived slight to myself or my family: an interruption of a story, uninterested friends, a rebuff of my son, a joke that hit a little too close. But it was all washed away with drinking. I was able to laugh at myself and ignore any slights.

The last day of my drinking we were having friends over for a barbeque. I was two beers into the evening when a friend asked me to write down a recipe. I couldn't read my own writing. I handed the recipe to him, hoping that I was just imagining that it was illegible. But he couldn't read it either. Even though I was drunk, I was aware of being terribly humiliated. It was time to stop.

This time I wanted to be sober, not just dry. I had to quit talking about not drinking. I just had to do it. I had images of all the good that would come of my sobriety. My health would be restored and I would lose the twenty pounds I had gained over all the years of drinking. I would be more productive in my free time and finally get those writing projects done, which would be rewarded with much success. I would attend parties and not worry about how I might embarrass myself.

I have been sober now for seven months. None of my dreams have come true yet. I am still twenty pounds overweight, though I don't have blotchy skin anymore, just wrinkles. I spend lots of what used to be hangover time working on writing and other projects. None have generated any more success than I was already experiencing. I am exercising just as little as before. Now when I attend parties, I am aware of all my missteps and inappropriate comments, which make me even more uncomfortable.

So why am I still sober? Because I hang onto the knowledge that I am not making myself sick. I am slowly gaining back my self-respect. I am learning to replace old habits with new ones. Each day I don't drink away a bit of my self-respect is a new and wonderful day.

I stay sober so that I can be there for myself and for my son, always, even when life is uncomfortable. In the mornings, when I write about being thankful for a new beginning, it is no longer with dread in my heart, but with hope. I want more than anything else to be fully awake for my life, and I know that if I don't take a drink, I am awake.

I am learning to love the taste of sobriety.

Diane Mierzwick taught middle school English in California for eighteen years. She is currently a literacy coordinator for parole education. She is married with a fourteen-year-old son, two dogs, three cats, one bird and thirteen fish.

Part II

I had to hide in my room, pretending to read while they were screaming downstairs...

It would have been better if he had robbed a store or stole a car...

I was powerless over my condition...

Daddy Hyde
Donna Veneto

I had a wonderful father. He was loving and caring and generally fun to be around. Everyone loved him, and he had many friends. But another father lived within him—Daddy Hyde—who caused pain, who would come around out of nowhere and destroy everything. My father's addiction to alcohol led him down a dark road to becoming Daddy Hyde, a journey he started as a teenager just having fun with his friends and ended as a broken man in a nursing home at age 44. Drink stole many things from him: mobility, livelihood, a normal life. It stole from the rest of us as well—a husband and father, a friend.

I cannot recall when I first knew that my father was an alcoholic, or even when I first learned what an alcoholic was. I knew from a very young age that he spent many nights away from home, "working late" as my mother told me, and that he had a violent temper. It is hard to say, however, exactly *when* I made the actual connection between his behavior and something outside of him, namely, alcohol. The perceptions of a child are so fresh, so young, and some things are now fuzzy in my mind. For example, I do not remember being aware of violence in the home at a young age, but I recently saw a home video that proves that I was aware of it at the time. On the video, my father was annoyed with my mother, who was playfully following him around with the video camera. Just before he slammed the door in her face, my young voice yells out, "Don't hit Mommy!" Yes, I was aware of Daddy Hyde.

I remember Daddy Hyde showing up on every Thanksgiving and Christmas. These holidays were supposed to be special and warm, yet they were filled with images of him cursing at and hitting my mother. The turkey never had much taste after that, the excitement over presents fell flat.

My younger sister and I sat in the back seat of our car many times while our mother drove frantically around the neighborhood, searching the bars for any sign of him. We always found him in one, and he was furious at having been found. In one instance, he came over to the car and tried to get in, but we were afraid and locked the doors. He pulled out his key while we were stuck at a red light, and I can still remember the absolute terror I felt. *What will he do if he gets to us?* Luckily the light turned green and my mother slammed her foot on the gas pedal, leaving him behind, key in hand.

The violence spread from my mother to my sister and me. There were many trips to the doctor—a sprained finger, headaches from having my head slammed into a wall… ahem, I mean, from accidentally bumping it, etc. I harbored such a great, dark secret from these doctors who looked at my father and me with knowing eyes. "Are you sure that's how it happened?" they would whisper. "Yes," I would answer, resolute. I had a fear of being taken away because this was my family, after all. I loved them. I loved my father, despite hating Daddy Hyde.

I have a distinct memory of standing in front of the Christmas tree, pouting, with my father at my back. "I'm going to go to A.A. I mean it this time," he said. "I'm going to stop drinking." I fiddled with an ornament as he spoke. "You always say that," I replied, with the arrogance and honesty of a child.

"I know, but this time it's for real. Do you forgive me?"

This episode would play itself out, over and over, but trips to A.A. meetings quickly became a cover for trips to the bar. After one particularly nasty episode, Daddy Hyde stormed out of the house, ostensibly leaving while remaining in the hallway, unseen. I turned to my mother, enraged. "He's not acting like a man! He's acting like a boy!" It was the strongest statement I could make at that age, with my limited vocabulary and undaunted respect for my father. At that moment, he re-entered, his eyes glassy and red. He looked me straight in the eye and said, "Donna, I heard what you said, and you are not my daughter anymore." Then he left, and I collapsed against my pillow, sobbing.

The secret was ours to keep and hide from the world. I was terrified that my friends would learn that my father had a drinking problem. (Little did I know that they, and the entire neighborhood, knew as much). My mother felt like a hypocrite every time they went to church, and when I was ten years old, they stopped going altogether for this very reason, despite having been extremely religious. She could no longer bear the Saturday night drinking binges and abuse directly followed by the fake "family in church" show that we put on each week.

The worst altercation between Daddy Hyde and me occurred when I was fourteen years old. I had become a rebellious teen in a very superficial sense: I went to school, got straight A's and didn't drink, do drugs or have sex, but I was incredibly disrespectful in the home. I lashed out at my parents, the anger from my childhood spilling over into everyday spats and issues. At times, I was downright venomous.

One such time was a weekday evening when my mother insisted that my father take me to my aunt's house to spend the night. Daddy Hyde took over and threw me out of the house. When he came out to get me, I ran from him, shouting angry words while maintaining a safe distance. After he went back inside, I sat on our front step and wept. Suddenly the door opened and the chase was on. I ran down the block until he caught me by my hair and dragged me to the car. He shoved me in, bumping my head and leaving an enormous lump. He sped through the streets like a maniac, and although I eyed the door when we stopped at red lights, I was too afraid to defy him. When we arrived at my aunt's apartment, I frantically searched for a chance to escape. He knew what I was thinking and smacked my face hard, saying, "You want to run?"

To be fair, there was much laughter and love and fun in my relationship with my father, yet how can one forget the actions of Daddy Hyde? I am haunted still by the effects of alcohol on my father, and the monster he became because of it. I always wondered if it was a disease or a choice. Could he be blamed or not? To this day, I am unsure. Sometimes I feel terribly sorry for him, wondering what it would be like to have an addiction that's so strong that you are forced to watch yourself harm your family and repeat travesty after travesty, over and over again. Other times I think, as I did then, that he could have tried harder. He could have made A.A. work. He could have done something, but he didn't.

Fast forward. I am twenty years old, sitting at the computer, writing a paper on Thoreau for my English class. It is 8:00 o'clock on a Wednesday evening. The house is quiet. My father has been playing with my younger sisters. He is visiting: my mother has demanded a separation, and he lives with his mother, who looks the other way after drunken escapades. Just weeks ago he attempted to kick my mother down the stairs. He has a new anger management technique—putting his hands around her neck to choke her. Tonight my father is over, not Daddy Hyde. There has been no violence, no evil. He asks my mother if he can spend the night.

My mother looks around at her daughters, knowing that she sets an example with every action she takes. She politely refuses, saying, "I don't think it's a good idea." He becomes angry. She relents, but his pride has been wounded and he storms out. "Bye

Donna," he says while passing me to the door. "Bye Dad," I say without looking up.

In the middle of the night, at around 2 A.M., a banging on the door stirs me from my slumber. My sister answers the door, my mother comes downstairs. The detectives step through the door and tell us that he has been in a car accident. I am puzzled; he did not leave in a car. "Is it serious?" my mother asks. "Ma'am, we wouldn't be here," the detective answers grimly.

In the end, my father is no longer an alcoholic. He is a quadriplegic. After leaving our home in the early evening, he went to a local bar and drank for hours straight, then staggered out into the street without looking. He was nearly killed when he was struck by a speeding car. He now lives in a nursing home where he can do nothing but watch television and depend on others for basic things like eating, brushing his teeth or scratching an itch. He is brave, but often depressed. He misses his home and his family, and he has profusely apologized for the things that Daddy Hyde has done. There is no chance of recovery from this. Alcohol has destroyed his life.

Donna Veneto is a college senior majoring in literature, as well as a freelance writer. She has worked in communications, marketing, and in the art world in Europe. Her work has been published in the *Austin American-Statesman* and various magazines and websites. She enjoys reading, long walks and spending time with good friends, and her goal is to make a difference in people's lives through her writing.

(continued from page 10)

What Are Alcohol Use Disorders?

Alcohol use disorders (AUDs) are clinical syndromes that include withdrawal, abuse and dependence (also known as alcoholism), as well as disorders that are caused by the effects of alcoholism such as dementia, depression, and anxiety. However, while these disorders are defined by a cluster of symptoms occurring over time, a single episode of alcohol misuse, even if it does not meet the clinical criteria used to define a "disorder," can lead to unwanted, negative outcomes for the drinker, his family or society. For example, Mason, a usually well behaved high school senior, got drunk, stole his parents' car, wrecked it and suffered severe injuries. Jenny, a sophomore in college who seldom touched alcohol, drank too much at a party and ended up having sex with another student she met only that night. She later tested positive for a sexually transmitted disease, something that never would have happened had she not drunk to excess.

13.7 % of all adults in the United States suffer from alcohol abuse or dependence disorders. Despite changing trends in substance use in our culture, AUDs are the most common substance problems in our country: there are more than twice as many adults with alcohol disorders than all other drug use disorders combined (including opioids, cocaine, marijuana, and other drugs of abuse).

(continued on page 38)

King Alcohol and His Loyal Subject

Tracy Alverson

My father never beat me. He never beat my mother. He never beat my brother. In fact, most times, he didn't do much of anything but sit at the kitchen counter slumped over a chipped mug filled with expensive scotch (or cheap vodka, depending on the bank account) in his bathrobe at five in the afternoon crying or staring blankly at the T.V.

I adored him growing up; he was a brilliant man and would have died for me if I had asked. We lived in a beautiful house in a great neighborhood and my backyard had woods to play in and sheep to feed through a white picket fence. I had frilly dresses to wear to family occasions, and every Christmas I'd gasp at the number of presents under our tree. I don't remember things going sour, and I don't remember seeing my father with anything other than a glass of Scotch in his hand at the end of a workday.

At nine years old I knew my father had a problem and I knew life was going to change. "He just won't admit he's an alcoholic," my mother would say. I knew she was right. Fifteen years later, when I visited him in the hospital as he lay in a pool of his own piss and blood, he declared, "There's no such thing as alcoholism. I just drink alcoholically."

I'd always assumed alcoholics lived off cheap vodka and slept under park benches; they beat their wives and children and ran off with prostitutes. My dad had a master's degree and $400 suits. He liked Scotch, sure, but he was a *businessman*: they were allowed to drink because they had *stress*.

Two days after hearing my mother say those words, we attended a Christmas party where my father had one too many drinks and threw my mother off the porch. Two months after that, my family had an intervention and I had to hide in my room, pretending to read while they were screaming downstairs. A year after that, we lost the mortgage on our beautiful home and my parents filed for bankruptcy.

Six years later we were living in a new home, this one featuring a sun room filled with my father's model sailboats and first edition books. He was working from home now and during our first summer in the house we built a rock garden together in the backyard. I was in high school and my parents encouraged me to take advance placement classes and join swim team. I was bored with school and doing all the things teenagers do, smoking pot and sneaking into movies, skipping classes and sitting in diners for entire afternoons while my parents thought I was in Art History. My father wasn't drinking, and he was on an anti-depressant which made him function like a human being again. It was amazing. We were a normal American family.

By my sophomore year of high school, he was drinking again. In the fall, we began to notice him going into the basement more often than usual. My father spent hours down there, going through boxes of junk we had accumulated and drinking vodka. Vodka might not smell but anyone could tell he'd been sipping when he stumbled into the kitchen for dinner at night with glassy eyes and a silly smile on his face. By Christmas he was up to a bottle a day, and everyone knew what he was up to, but he'd never admit it. During our holiday party he made crude jokes and hit on my mother's friends. I was embarrassed by this brazen man who claimed to be my dad. This man, who would normally be hiding in the kitchen helping my mom prepare cheese platters. We knew it wouldn't be long until he hit his umpteenth rock bottom, and he did that spring.

I remember that evening so clearly I get chills writing about it now. I was upstairs, watching a movie about Anne Frank when I heard the crash. Then I heard my mother crying for help, instructing me to call 911. When you are the child of an alcoholic parent, you live for these moments, any crash, any bang or scream and your hand is poised on the phone ready to call for help. I blubbered to the woman on the phone, I might have said my dad has finally lost it, he's going to kill my mom The phone was taken away from me and I was left rocking myself in the hallway, wondering what had happened. The police arrived; I peeked at them from the balcony upstairs. A few minutes after that, the paramedics were called. I saw my mother sobbing, being questioned. My father saw me as he was being wheeled out. Our eyes locked. His head was cut open on one side and his clothes and the blanket he was wrapped in were covered in blood. A police officer saw me staring and ordered me to go to my room, told me not to watch. I heard one of them say, "It looks like someone got murdered down here."

Family members were called to stay with me; my mother was being held for questioning. My aunt explained that my mother had snapped and taken my father's vodka bottle and smashed him over the head with it, kept hitting him even after he fell down and begged her to stop. Why, I asked? Why would she do that to my dad? My aunt was quiet for a while, then she explained he had threatened to hurt her, hurt me, and she wanted him to stop, wanted it to end once and for all.

My father went to rehab, his third, after this incident, one of those smarmy places that cost half your life savings, an estate nestled in the middle of the woods. With my dad gone, life was pleasant and I remember we went out to dinner at the Ground Round a lot and I drank endless raspberry iced teas and ate endless platters of French fries. A few months later it was time to pick him up and I volunteered to go with my mother because I was curious about rehab; they seemed like mini vacations to me and I expected my father to be tanned and fit, cured of his disease.

Once in the facility I became wary of the smiles being sent my way. Happy people make me nervous, and even though I was fifteen years old I hid behind my mother while she filled out paperwork. People came up to me to tell me how my father had helped them, inspired them, how brilliant he was and how much he had changed. *I don't believe you* I chanted over and over in my head, giving them the middle finger with my mind while we waited for the man of the hour to appear. When he did show he looked pale and taut. He smiled at me sadly as we were ushered into the social worker's office. A.A. meetings were required, therapy and medication required, all things my father hated and would refuse within two weeks of his release. I wanted to smack the shit out of the polyester-clad social worker but I sat there and nodded along with my dad, like daughter like father, and when the woman turned to me and said, "and what can you do," I kept nodding like she hadn't asked me a question.

What can I do? Well lady, I can sit up at night wondering if my dad's daydreaming about tumblers filled with Scotch. I can pretend that entire years of my life didn't happen, and that my dad didn't punch walls and fall down stairs when he should have been helping me learn algebra. I can stop obsessing about the smell of his breath and wonder if it's mouthwash or booze and I can rest easy and not study his every move wondering when he's going to start drinking again. A fifteen year old, lady, cannot stop her forty-year-old father from drinking himself to death, don't put that responsibility on me.

But she already had. I had to save my father.

Years passed and life continued to crumble apart. I saw him through three more years of rehab and I wanted so badly for him to get better that my heart hurt. My mother decided to leave my dad, and deep down inside, I knew it was about time, but I couldn't leave his side. We lost our house: he wasn't working and he was drinking again and my mother found an apartment down the road that she couldn't afford. I stayed with my father, knowing we would get evicted together and that when he hit another bottom I would scoop him up and cater to his every need. In June, I was reading in the sunroom when I heard him fall to the floor. He was having a seizure. He couldn't afford booze and hadn't had a drink in a few hours. I walked in and held his head, dialed 911 and told the woman my father was withdrawing from alcohol and to send an ambulance. They knew where to go.

The following year we were out of our pretty suburban house and living in a rented space at the beach. He'd been sober for three months. But I ended up calling my mom crying one night, asking if I could come live with her because Dad was drinking again and this time I couldn't help him, this time he'd gone too far. I moved in with her and we began to patch things up as a family, and I tried to forget about my father who by the end of the summer was living in a motel.

I landed in the hospital myself that fall and the day I came out Mom was picking up Chinese for dinner when the doorbell rang. It was my father; he was crawling up the stairs to our apartment, slurring his words and asking why I was in the hospital. He had driven two hours from his motel to our house and I wondered if he killed anyone on the way. I locked myself in my bedroom, sobbing to my mother that he had come back, and I called 911 from my room because I wanted him out, I needed him out. He was drinking out of a brown paper bag when they came and it took four men to heave him out of the house because he couldn't walk. We found out a few weeks later he had stolen a pocket full of our jewelry to pawn to buy booze. My father has taken everything from us over the years.

Two years have passed since that night and he's only gotten worse. A social worker found him in a motel room one night, covered in his own urine, feces and blood, and he was in the hospital for almost two months because he was emaciated and near death. He has been diagnosed with cancer. I was the only one who visited him in the hospital, the only one who went to the hotel room to clean up the blood and throw out his bottles (I found close to fifty).

I choose not to see my father very often these days. There are times of normalcy, and if asked to reflect on my teenhood I will rave. I will speak of the vacations when we rented a boat and sailed on Lake Wallenpaupack. I will describe the hiking trips my father took us on, where he explained what every plant was. I will tell of the time my father bought me my first 35mm camera and drove me all over New Jersey to take pictures of the sunrise over the mountains or the sunset at the beach. "Your dad sounds pretty amazing," everyone will say to me now that I'm twenty-two. And I will answer, "But I hate him."

I am starting a life of my own, and he doesn't want help. He knows he drinks too much but he has justified all the times he's stolen from us, threatened my mother, come close to physically harming one of his children. I choose instead to live with the pleasant memories I have. It's not my fault my father wants to die and is slowly killing himself with the bottle. It is not my fault that he won't listen to me, and the only regret I have is helping him on the path of destruction.

The author resides with her fiancé, their cat and several hundred books in Staten Island, New York. An expectant mother, she spends her time working on blogs and essays, pet sitting and arts and crafts. She has lived with alcoholism her entire life and contributes this essay in the hope it will help people understand that they are not alone.

A Parent's Trial
Anne Pascale

Entering the laundry room, I gaze at the shelf full of my son Michael's old clothes, all neatly folded. They bring back memories of a delightful golden-haired boy. Not the one now in jail. What happened? I resent this imposter while fearing for his safety. My efforts to help him are futile, his behavior an unstoppable cyclone. An alcoholic like his father, my ex-husband.

He lies to me so successfully, because I desperately wish to believe his tales as household objects disappear, including his prize electric guitar—sold to buy liquor. The circumstantial evidence defeats optimism. I'm stalked by the uncertainty of never knowing the full truth.

I clutch his once-favorite jean shirt, an embroidered Looney Tunes design on its back. Definitely uncool by his present standards. It contrasts sharply with his three felony charges for selling drugs. Tears fall along familiar pathways across my careworn face. While infomercials promise that informed youth don't consume drugs, I know it's not so. No protective shield exists. Hereditary influences trump my crying, my yelling and pleading. He began drinking at fourteen, his first arrest was at fifteen, a dropout by sixteen. Two stints of probation, community service and various counselors have not put an end to his destructive actions.

I put his shirt on, wrapping it tightly around me. Uncontrollable sobs begin. I admit to relief: at least I know where he is. No tracing the caller ID. No pounding on unknown doors at 7 A.M. No wondering who is entering my home—my son or this irritable, self-absorbed, depressed stranger.

I've abandoned examining his thought processes. His high tolerance tricks him into believing he's problem-free. He crashes as soon as his drinking stops. I'm ashamed, thinking his behavior stems from a lack of morals, like his father before him, but I know physiology and genetics determine his unfortunate reaction to alcohol. It's a disease, not an emotional weakness.

Traumatic memories flash into my mind, of him in handcuffs before the judge. I'm stricken with fear over what jail will teach a boy playing in a man's world. Still clasping his shirt, I walk to his bedroom. Total disarray: furniture upturned, cushions taken apart, ceiling panels removed: debris of a desperate search by family for his hidden pharmacy... a rainbow of pills, household containers filled with alcohol. Drugs. In our home. Who *is* this child? Grief pours through me. If I had done something different, would he be the same? Accepting that I have no control is a major hurdle, too high to jump some days. It's easier imagining I'm in command, similar to believing in Santa Claus. A constant struggle ensues between dread over what may happen and anger at his actions. But my son was forgiving:

"This is not about you," he declared. "I did this, not you."

"What if I had dragged you to court and placed you residentially?"

"We'd have no relationship now," he said simply. "You're a good parent," he added.

Love and wrath battled inside me. The lawyer tells us it would have been better if he had robbed a store or stolen a car: the judge would see him more as a user than as a dealer. What does this mean? If you blow it big time, the authorities have more compassion? I worry about his physical safety. Maturity stunted by drugs; a fourteen-year-old in an eighteen-year-old's body. In prison.

The father fights against and undermines my efforts to force Michael into treatment. He alternates between being his buddy and projecting his own failures. Having a propensity for drink, my ex started in earnest following Michael's birth. Money went for liquor, not groceries or medical expenses, eventually leading to bankruptcy. He quit seven years later because of blackouts. Stopped cold, but his unpredictable behavior remains, alternating between self-pity and paranoia, between avoiding responsibility and belligerence.

My ex-husband's vagueness for details and refusal to be accountable are reborn in my son. Enough of cheap apologies, I await a different ending. No release from jail unless he agrees to treatment. I will do what's in Michael's best interest—be a parent and pray. I remove his shirt, drying my tears on its sleeve. I fold it, placing it back on the pile. I look again at the neatly stacked clothes. Maybe the pile is more symbolic of things to come; a restructuring of Mike's choices. Maybe the fabric of our life can still come clean. Some stains will fade while others will be ignored and forgotten.

Anne Pascale is a therapist by trade, a parent for life. Her work has been published in regional magazines and in an anthology on travel, and it has been read on National Public Radio. She currently directs a day treatment program for emotionally disturbed adolescents.

(continued from page 28)

What Causes Alcohol Problems?

Many social, psychological and even biological factors interact to contribute to the prevalence of AUDs. Social factors include the wide availability of alcohol, pressure to drink by others, the influence of family and friends and the cultural acceptance of alcohol use or intoxication. Psychological factors include the use of alcohol to cope with and manage stress and emotions, psychiatric disorders such as depression or post-traumatic stress disorder, and personality traits such as thrill seeking or shyness. Biological factors include a genetic vulnerability to the substance (alcohol problems run in families), how a person metabolizes alcohol, the individual's inherent physical tolerance to the drug, and the abuse of other drugs by the individual. (Many people with AUDs also use, abuse or are dependent on other substances such as opioids, stimulants, cannabis, nicotine, hallucinogens or depressant drugs, all of which negatively affect the course of alcoholism and recovery from it. In addition, nearly 40% of individuals with AUDs also have a co-existing psychiatric illness, such as mood, anxiety, psychotic, personality, or eating disorders, which can also complicate the recovery from alcoholism.) Genetics plays a role as well: deficiencies in the body's natural "reward system," which creates feelings of pleasure when people take part in enjoyable activities, may lead some people to self-medicate with alcohol in order to feel "normal."

Addictive drugs, like alcohol, work on the same part of the brain that causes activities such as eating and having sex to be pleasurable. Called the *reward pathway* or the *mesolimbic dopamine pathway*, this area runs from the base of the brain to the very front of the brain behind the eyes. It evolved in human beings to make eating food and engaging in sexual reproduction rewarding and important so that we engage in these behaviors repeatedly: regular food consumption helps the health of the individual and engaging in reproduction ensures the continuation of the species. Addictive drugs, such as alcohol, stimulate this same pathway. In fact, it is the stimulation of the reward pathway that makes alcohol *habituating*, or addictive, for some individuals.

The more frequently this system is stimulated by alcohol, the more the use of alcohol assumes a central importance in the individual's life and the more a person "wants" to use alcohol. Over time, the use of alcohol becomes of central importance in the life of the alcoholic, while friends, family, loved ones, sex, food, sports, hobbies, and other naturally rewarding activities become less important. This "hijacking" of the brain's reward pathway ultimately results in dependence on alcohol. Understanding the effects of alcohol on the reward pathway helps us to better understand why it is so difficult to stop using alcohol once a person has become addicted: when an individual stops drinking, the brain has to "reset" itself, so that the natural rewards once again stimulate the reward pathway as strongly as alcohol did in the past. This process takes time, which may help explain why some alcoholics relapse—their brains have not had enough time to adjust to sober living.

The other important elements of alcohol dependence, *tolerance* and *withdrawal*, can also be traced to the effect on the brain of repeated alcohol use. The brain normally engages in very delicate biological processes. Alcohol alters normal brain function and throws these processes out of balance. But the brain is remarkable organ. It can adjust itself so that it gradually returns to a normal level of functioning despite alcohol's presence and impact on its natural physiology. This process of adjustment or adaptation by the brain to repeated or continuous exposure to alcohol is known as *tolerance*. Tolerance can be either a reduction in the effect of alcohol on the brain over time or the need for higher doses of alcohol to achieve the same pleasurable effect.

Alcohol withdrawal occurs when the brain has adjusted its own physiology to the presence of alcohol, and the amount of the alcohol present is then reduced or removed. The brain then has to undo all of the adaptive changes it had previously made. The symptoms produced by this "undoing" of changes are known as *withdrawal syndrome*.

(continued on page 49)

A Sister's Regret
Gloria Raskin

Tomorrow is my brother's birthday. If Arthur were alive, he would be sixty-two years old. He should be alive. His life should have turned out differently. But he died of cirrhosis of the liver almost eight years ago, brought on by continual drinking. At the time of his death I had so much resentment toward him and so little understanding of his problems. But it was not in my power to make him stop drinking. He made his own choices. Everyone urged him to attend Alcoholics Anonymous meetings, but he laughed at the suggestions. He laughed at everyone who did not need alcohol to cope with life.

There was a six-year age difference between us that created a canyon of separateness never filled during our lives. Resentment probably grew before love did. I wonder why it was difficult to love my brother when he was alive; I think about how much I love him now. As I write this, the tears come, and I wish I could relive my life, somehow do it over again and be kinder, gentler, and sweeter to my only sibling. My husband reminds me that I was very protective toward my brother when we were younger, but I remember only the harsher, more recent actions. I do recall taking him for his driving test, and asking my boyfriend, now my husband, to do "boy" things with him, such as ball playing and scouting. These were the things my father never did with Arthur, either through choice or timing. My father was a hard worker, and when he came home he was more than content to sit in his chair and read the newspaper, or play with his stamp collection.

Arthur was twice-divorced with three children. The last divorce was a bitter one and it left him lonely and lost. He took to drinking to deal with the pain, and eventually lost his job as a salesman and moved in with our mother. Mother was having problems of her own, coping with widowhood and medical issues. Mother walked to the laundry to get Arthur's shirts and cooked his meals, which often went uneaten, and begged the neighborhood liquor store not to sell him alcohol. She also frequently watered down his drinks, which led to violent confrontations. She complained to me constantly about my brother and sought my help in "fixing" the problem. There seemed to be a continual war between Arthur and Mother, and it fueled my resentment of him even more. Eventually, the fighting escalated between them and became physical. Orders of protection were filed and Arthur spent a night or two in jail. I was horrified at this and I wanted to literally kill my brother. Why was he behaving like this? Why was he making life so difficult for my mother and me? Why was everybody in the family involved in this situation?

I gave Arthur money from my mother's account on the condition that he leave her apartment and find another place to live. My husband met him in the city and gave him $5,000 in cash to get him on his feet again. We felt as if we were making a positive step in the family's relationships until we got home that evening and listened to a message from Arthur on our answering machine that deteriorated from sincere gratitude to wild accusations and incredible curses. He had used part of the money for alcohol.

My family wanted to try an intervention to get Arthur into a rehab facility. We spoke to a representative of a nearby institution, who told us that my mother had to change the locks to her apartment so that Arthur would be forced to stay at the rehab. This plan was abandoned when my mother refused. If only I could have made Mother understand that she was enabling Arthur to continue his drinking, and that forcing him into a healing facility might have saved him. The shame I should have felt that evening was buried by anger and annoyance, but looking back, I wonder why I couldn't have reversed matters then. If I had, maybe Arthur would be alive.

Arthur continued drinking. He eventually ended up in a city-run hospital, where he waited to die. He was unconscious most of the time. When I was told Arthur was going to die, I did not believe it. When the time actually came, I mechanically performed all the tasks necessary, including supporting my mother through the most difficult thing a mother can ever do: bury a child.

The only other person closely involved with my brother was Paul, his son from Arthur's first marriage. Paul got married shortly before Arthur became seriously ill. I remember my brother at Paul's small wedding ceremony, joking that it's easy to get married but difficult to get divorced. His lame joke was inappropriate at the time, and I was relieved when he disappeared from the reception. Paul had a difficult time accepting me into his life because he was raised to believe that I was his father's enemy. Thankfully, we have been able to put this aside, and I am now a small part of Paul's life. I know Arthur would have been proud of the man Paul has become: responsible, hard-working, caring, a good father. I know that, at one point in his life, my brother had all those traits too. Maybe Arthur's spirit lives on in his son.

Gloria Raskin is a wife, mother and grandmother of two little girls. She was born and raised in Brooklyn, New York, graduated from Brooklyn College and taught kindergarten for four years. She left teaching to raise her family and later received a master's degree in Special Education from Hofstra University in Hempstead, Long Island. She returned to teaching and retired several years ago. She now devotes her time to her grandchildren and her writing.

Two Mothers
Lisa Dordal

I had two mothers growing up: a daytime mother and a nighttime mother. My daytime mother was lively, smart, clear-eyed and beautiful. She had a certain style, particularly in her younger days. I remember seeing her in an old family movie where, for a moment, I thought I was watching a movie star. There she was, walking nonchalantly down the streets of some European city wearing a short brown bob and a sleeveless two-piece pantsuit that was all the rage in the Seventies. Her gait was spirited, her smile broad and uncontainable.

My daytime mother loved seeing new places and meeting new people. Like when she drove my three siblings and me down to Mexico in 1977 and made a point of avoiding all the hot-spot tourist places. We stayed in Mexican hotels, not American Hiltons or Holiday Inns, the kind of hotels you had to take narrow, winding roads to get to. Her love of adventure was matched by a strong sense of social justice. After World War II she spent two summers in Germany helping to rebuild a church in a town that had been ravaged by the war. Later, in the demonstration-filled days of the Sixties, she attended one peace rally after another in Chicago's Grant Park, peace necklace and all.

My nighttime mother was not as enjoyable to be around. She was sluggish and blurry-eyed. Her speech was thickly slurred and, at times, you could almost see the fog that surrounded her. My nighttime mother's drink of choice was the Manhattan, made of bourbon and vermouth, and always on the rocks. She would start drinking around five while she was preparing dinner and would continue drinking, one after another, until she went to bed at eleven. My bedroom was just off the back stairs, so every evening I would listen to the creak of the stairs and the clank of ice against the inside of her mug as she made her way up for the evening one slow, careful step after another. I would hear her call out to me when she reached the top of the stairs. "Good night" and "I love you," she would say, as cheerfully as her drunkenness allowed. Sometimes, later on in the evening, I would hear her go back downstairs to the butler's pantry to refill her mug. She didn't always refill her drink downstairs, though, because she had several secret stashes upstairs.

My mother's drinking continued like this until she retired at the age of sixty-six. She had been a family counselor for over thirty years and never had any intention of retiring. But she was asked to—budget cuts or some such reason. And that was the beginning of the end for my daytime mother. The line between daytime and nighttime became blurred during my mother's retirement years. There was no real reason for her to get up anymore. She could sleep as late as she wanted and consequently she could drink all through the night, something painfully brought home to me when I called her one morning a little after ten. I had been expecting to hear my daytime mother's voice, clear-eyed and chipper. Instead I heard the slurred words of my nighttime mother.

Five years later, my mother died.

At the age of thirty, six years before my mother died, I was well on my way to following in her footsteps. I had been married for five years and even though we didn't have kids yet, we were planning to start the "settling down" phase of our married life. I seemed to have it all: husband, house, long summer vacations and season tickets to the symphony. But my relationship with alcohol had never been a healthy one. I was fourteen years old the first time I got drunk. I don't remember many details of the incident, but I do remember the way I felt on the inside once the fog kicked in: warm and invincible. Like nothing could ever hurt me. Throughout high school and college I continued to drink, but rarely in front of my parents. It was usually at parties, with friends. Vodka or whiskey, sipped straight from the bottle. I didn't drink often enough to become physically addicted, but when I did drink, it was never in moderation.

My marriage ended abruptly. Never in my life had I felt so alone. It was as if God were purposely directing pain towards me. Out of my anger and despair I screamed, but heard nothing in return. Nothing but silence, silence and more silence.

Ironically, it was out of this silence, in the waiting for an answer, that my sense of wonder about the God against whom my anger was directed began to grow. For in the process of acknowledging my anger towards God, I was simultaneously acknowledging and passionately embracing the existence of my relationship with Him, and I began to feel a closeness to God for the first time in my life. Had I not experienced such a radical transformation of identity, I have little doubt that, in addition to following in my daytime mother's footsteps, I would someday have followed in my nighttime mother's footsteps as well.

But when my marriage ended, I lost my taste for alcohol. I lost my taste for anything that made me feel foggy or not quite me since, for the first time in my life, I felt *real*: filled with love not only for myself but for God as well. At her wake three days after she died, what struck me most was that my mother no longer smelled of alcohol. And as people from all corners of her life came to share stories about my mother—wonderfully uplifting stories about my daytime mother—I realized that my mother was free now at long, long last, and so was I.

Lisa Dordal lives in Nashville, Tennessee. She received a master's degree in Divinity from Vanderbilt University Divinity School, where she was the recipient of the Saint James Academy Award, the William A. Newcomb Prize, and the Luke-Acts Prize. Her writing has appeared in *Alive Now*, *Theology Today* and *The Vanderbilt Review*. She is the author of a memoir, *The Wild in Me Wears Purple*.

(continued from page 40)

What Are the Classification of Alcohol Use Disorders?

There are five generally accepted types AUDs, and they are classified by the physical and psychological symptoms exhibited by the affected individual:

Alcohol intoxication. This is a reversible syndrome caused by recent alcohol use. Physiological signs include slurred speech, the loss of physical coordination, an unsteady gait, *nystagmus*, or involuntary eye movement, flushed face, impairment in memory or attention, or stupor or coma. Behavioral or psychological signs may include inappropriate behavior, mood swings, impaired judgment, or impaired functioning at school, work, or in the family. The effects of alcohol intoxication may last hours and put the person at risk for accidents, medical problems or complications.

Alcohol withdrawal. Withdrawl is caused by reducing or stopping alcohol use following a period of heavy and prolonged drinking. Symptoms of alcohol withdrawal include two or more of the following symptoms: sweating or elevated blood pressure, increased hand tremor, insomnia, nausea or vomiting, transient hallucinations, agitation, anxiety or seizures.

Alcohol abuse. This involves a maladaptive pattern of alcohol use leading to distress or impairment with at least one of four of the following symptoms occurring within a 12-month period: a failure to fulfill obligations at home, work or school, recurrent substance use in hazardous situations, recurrent legal problems, or continued substance use despite the persistence of problems caused by such use. Abuse does not include withdrawal, tolerance or compulsive use; it is repeated use that includes only harmful consequences.

Alcohol dependence (also called alcoholism). This pattern of alcohol use leads to distress or impairment with at least three or more of the following symptoms occurring within a 12-month period: increased or decreased tolerance; withdrawal symptoms or using substances to avoid or relieve alcohol withdrawal; the loss of control over or the inability to reduce use; spending a great deal of time to obtain or recover from alcohol; giving up or reducing important activities because of alcohol use; and continued use despite being aware of a persistent or recurrent physical or psychological problem caused or exacerbated by alcohol use.

Alcohol induced mood, anxiety, and psychotic-induced disorders. These are prominent psychiatric symptoms caused by the physiological effects of alcohol. Alcohol use can contribute to all types of psychiatric symptoms, especially in those who are dependent.

(continued on page 56)

The Healing Power of Truth
Karen W. Waggoner

No one recovers from alcoholism. It is a chronic disease that cannot be cured. Everyone who has alcoholism will die an alcoholic. But I do not have to die of drink, nor must I waste my life in the despair that my condition causes if untreated. If I arrest my disease, I can thrive for my full lifespan and receive a gift of understanding that many others never achieve.

I didn't know any of this fifteen years ago, when I was a fifty-year-old English teacher of unfailing moral character. I had been faithful to my husband for thirty years and had not had a drink in a bar for ten or more years. I sang in the church choir until I gave it up because my nerves were too bad to tolerate public performance. As far as I know, none of my friends knew that I drank to excess because I hid it so well. I never considered drinking in the morning or at school. At home, I concealed my bottles and my drinking habits from others by withdrawing more and more into my own room and away from my family's expectations.

My social life was buried under subterfuge. Because I suspected that the local store clerks counted my purchases, I drove long distances to buy liquor. I rarely drank when I was with friends; I did without a drink until I got home where I could indulge my habit in private. As a result, it got to the point where I seldom accepted invitations to go anywhere, and I never entertained.

I just could not grasp the truth of my condition until I reached the point where I could no longer hide from myself. On a trip to visit our son in a distant city, I waited to drink until he and my husband were gone for the day. Then I spent that day alone in the hotel room, getting quietly and completely drunk. Not long after that, my husband called me from the airport because his car had failed, and he needed me to pick him up. I was already impaired. Of course I couldn't tell him that, so I drove to the terminal in profound terror of having an accident or being caught by the police. I'll never forget how frightened I was.

My shame was devastating, and my isolation deepened until I became afraid to answer the phone most evenings. I was sure someone would detect my drunkenness. Perhaps the worst of all the misery was the realization that in order to enjoy my grandchildren, as well as to care for them adequately, I had to abstain from alcohol while they were in my home. Their visits became ordeals of painful withdrawal while I waited to mix a drink.

For many of us alcoholics, especially those "high bottom" drunks like me who haven't yet lost everything, reaching the point of facing reality doesn't arrive quickly. It isn't as if we commit violent crimes, are sentenced to prison, and find our lives destroyed. No, we continue to function for years and years, gradually acknowledging to ourselves that we have a problem with alcohol but are too ashamed, too powerless, and too ignorant to do anything about it. Meanwhile, the erosion of our families, our careers, and our self-esteem continues. I was able to observe my withdrawal from my grandchildren, from relationships with my children and from friendships, not to mention my marriage. It wasn't until many years later that I saw clearly the utter selfishness of my life as it deteriorated.

The arrival of truth was a miracle, the culmination of years of small realizations. I am convinced that the hand of divine Providence, logic, and God pushed me toward the telephone on a snowy February morning in 1991. It was then that I began the process of getting acquainted with my disease. Too busy and too proud to take time off from work, I did not go to a formal treatment course but attended many meetings where I generally did little but listen. Over a period of weeks, then months, and finally years, I learned that I must surrender to my powerlessness over alcohol not just once but every hour, every day, every week, every month until it became a part of my psyche. Even then, I reinforced my conviction on a regular basis by associations with sober friends. Still later, my greatest happiness grew from my contact with many young people in early stages of treatment. Mentoring them allows me to explore my own story and my beliefs with ever-expanding understanding.

My disease, my condition, my chemical makeup, maybe even my character make it impossible for me to resist the ease and comfort that alcohol brings to me. We who suffer from alcoholism love the effect of drinking more than we love ourselves, our jobs, our families, or our integrity. There are very few hard rules about recovery from alcoholism, but the first rule is that we face our defeat in order to arrive at freedom from the dominance of alcohol. I had to reach the point where I could not live without drinking, and yet could not continue to drink. I had to accept that I am different from the neighbors who can take a drink or two with impunity. I am different from the neighbors who don't care one way or another about having a drink. Despite the fact that I loathed being different, I made that life or death decision. I chose, and choose, to live.

I was also forced to make some other brutal choices early in my recovery. First, I had to decide to change anything in my life that seemed to be part of the problem. I convinced myself that sometimes I drank to escape from my long marriage and my husband, who had some problems of his own. I even decided that I would end the marriage if it meant I could live without drinking. I likewise recognized that the stress of my teaching career gave me an excuse to drink by giving me the habitual need to relax, calm down, change my focus, or go to sleep. I postponed acting on either conclusion, heeding the advice of my new friends and counselors who admonished me not to make drastic changes in my life until I could be sure my thinking was no longer clouded and confused by alcohol. They cautioned me to wait until I was certain that my emotions had stabilized. All of this took considerable time. Eventually I realized that both my husband and my career were not the problem; I was the problem.

Years later, and with an ongoing education in treating my alcoholism, I remain convinced that admitting defeat is the most crucial understanding for me. If I do not accept my powerlessness over alcohol every single day, every hour of the day, I cannot be confident of my future. I have repeated this truth often enough that it is a part of my body, my soul, my very self, so that actually dwelling on it is not necessary any more.

Nearly every experience involving alcohol helps me to reinforce the truth I have worked so hard to accept. For example, on a recent drive through Missouri, I entered a gas station-convenience store where liquor was sold. On my way to the ladies room, I saw an enormous display of gin bottles catching the light and glowing with remarkable allure. I slowed my pace but continued on my errand. When I returned to the car I asked my husband if he had noticed the display. He said he had not. Am I the alcoholic? You bet!

Only a few years after I accepted being "different" from other people, my husband and I retired. We moved away from the city and took up a new lifestyle in a small town in the South. Since that time, I have completed and published the novel I began more than twenty years ago. I continue to write daily and to work with the writing group I formed after I retired. I have been a volunteer for a local treatment center for alcoholics and addicts for nearly ten years and often have the pleasure of working with young women one to one. Sometimes I need to pinch myself to believe my good fortune.

I thank God daily that I did not have to accept a death sentence, nor cringe with guilt and fear. I accept my being different from others as a fact, and I go on with my life, understanding that I will always have alcoholism, but being different is sometimes a blessing.

Karen W. Waggoner is a retired high school English teacher, novelist, mother of two, grandmother of two and wife of a retired Navy chief. She holds an undergraduate degree from Stetson University and a graduate degree from the University of Connecticut. Her retirement has allowed her to finish a book, write and publish several shorter pieces, and make about a dozen quilts as well as volunteer to work with newcomers to alcohol and drug recovery. Her novel *On My Honor, A Navy Wife's Vietnam War*, was published in 2003.

(continued from page 50)

How Are Alcohol Problems Diagnosed?

AUDs are diagnosed by gathering information about the individual's alcohol use, problems and functioning and determining if the person meets the criteria for one of the disorders described above. Prior treatment records are reviewed and interviews are conducted of the person who drinks, her family members, her significant others and other treatment providers and/or the person who refers the drinker for an evaluation. Tests to help diagnose alcohol problems may include urinalysis, complete blood count with differential, blood chemistry, serology, and liver enzymes. Breath alcohol levels or blood alcohol concentration (BAC) tests provide objective measurements of the person's state of intoxication level and tolerance. Written questionnaires may also be used to assess current withdrawal symptoms for those physically addicted to alcohol. For example, the Clinical Alcohol Withdrawal Assessment (CIWA) scale is used to identify the severity of withdrawal symptoms and determine if medications are needed to manage these symptoms.

(continued on page 63)

Part III

"He's not an alcoholic," I tried to tell myself...

The worst part was the violence...

I prayed my **family** *would somehow make it through...*

May Day

Martha Deborah Hall

It's a beautiful May Day as we take the shore road to the hospital in Dad's maroon sedan. My older sister sits in front next to Dad, my twin sister next to me in back. We watch out the window as other children dive into high-tide waves. We keep driving until a sign on the right reads "Asylum Hill."

My mother is standing alone in the enclosed courtyard. We walk towards her. She does not say hello, does not stretch open her arms. The only sound is a hummingbird soothing itself on a trumpet vine. She walks away with my two sisters, leaves me behind with my dad. We follow silently.

When we leave, she hugs my sisters but not me. I think maybe she doesn't know I'm here. On the way home, my father tells us, "All she has to do to save this family is stop drinking."

In the back seat I remember all the liquor bottles I'd discovered around the house: on the side of her bed, buried under her gardenias in flower boxes, uncovered by the rain under tomato plants in her garden, under the lid to her upright piano, on the ground under her bedroom window. I was the one who told my father about the bottles. He already knew. I remember how our family money vanished in our efforts to save her… one-present birthdays, shabby clothes, burned-out light bulbs, used bicycles, broken dishes, yelling and screaming and suicide attempts. I remember gathering blueberries in the woods so my family could have something to eat.

That May Day is the last time I will see her—a blue spring day in that silent courtyard—the day seeds are planted to try to stop feeling and never look back.

Martha Deborah Hall is President of Amherst Historical Properties Real Estate, Ltd. in Manchester, New Hampshire. She has a Bachelor of Arts degree from Ohio Wesleyan and a master's degree from Columbia University. Her first chapbook, *Abandoned Gardens*, won the 2005 John & Miriam Morris Memorial Chapbook Competition and will be published this year. Her poems appear in many national journals, including *Bellowing Ark*, *Common Ground Review*, *Las Cruces*, *Old Red Kimono*, *Poet's Touchstone*, *Seldom Nocturne*, *Shemom* and *Watch the Eye*, and in the Nashua, New Hampshire *Poets Unbound* anthology, *Poems From the Cranberry Room*.

He's Not an Alcoholic
Mridu Khullar

"He's not an alcoholic," we thought, as he threw up over Mom's favorite couch cushions. This particular night, he'd had more than his usual quota. He stood up, legs wobbly from a combination of liquor, nausea and guilt. His lips curled and his brow wrinkled, but his eyes said he was sorry. Again.

"I don't drink because I like to; I drink because I'm sad," he kept repeating as we grew from children to teenagers, and from teenagers to adults. As a family of five that got along quite all right, I thought we were happy. But what did I know? I didn't understand the problems of adults; I didn't understand what made him the man he was. How could I possibly understand what went through his mind as he picked up the glass each night and headed off to drink alone?

He was a new man by day—the perfect father, the perfect husband and the perfect son. He was caring, considerate, and amidst the short bursts of temper, his love would shine through. But no one outside the family would have guessed what happened after the sun set each day—on the world and in our lives. Before long, he'd have a few in him, and he'd be a changed man. His speech slurred, he walked around purposelessly, his temper tantrums targeted anyone who crossed his path. He slept through cars back-firing on the street, short circuits in the house and even Mom's excruciating leg pains that, more than once, required calling in a doctor. The caring, nurturing father of the day was gone, and a desperate drowning man took his place.

"He's not an alcoholic," Mom would say, as she'd take the television remote control out of the refrigerator, where he'd put it in his half-awake state the night before. "He's just a little sad."

"He's not an alcoholic," I'd think, as I'd switch off the blaring television while he lay unconscious on the couch. I'd watch him every night through the crack in my door while I waited for him to snap out of his trance. Sometimes, he would, and then he'd make his way to his own bedroom upstairs where Mom slept, tired of waiting up for him.

"He's not an alcoholic," I convinced myself as he asked me for the second time when my college results would be out. I remembered having told him two days ago, but he'd been too much under the influence to hear what I'd said. Maybe the bottle was more important. Then again, maybe he was sad.

"He's not an alcoholic," we said each time he went out of control. And each time he shouted, screamed or threw verbal abuse our way. We defended him, covered up for him, and more than anything, protected him from discovering his own impotence.

"He's not an alcoholic," I whisper to myself as he slams the door shut. My mother sleeps on the couch downstairs. She no longer has the energy to combat him after a hard day at work. He lies in bed—retired, drunken, alone.

"He's not an alcoholic," I try to tell myself. This time though, I'm not so sure.

Mridu Khullar is a freelance journalist based in New Delhi, India, whose past work has been published in books, newspapers and magazines including *Marie Claire, ELLE, Chicken Soup for the Soul, World & I* and *The Times of India*, among many others.

(continued from page 56)

How Does One Know What Treatment Is Needed for An AUD?

Determining the proper treatment for an alcohol disorder depends on the unique problems and needs of the individual. The American Society on Addiction Medicine (ASAM) recommends that treatment decisions be based on a comprehensive assessment of six dimensions of functioning. This assessment determines the severity of the AUD and related medical or psychiatric disorders, which in turn determines the level of care needed. The assessment is conducted by a professional trained in addiction medicine (a physician, nurse, psychologist, social worker, counselor, or therapist). The six dimensions of the ASAM assessment are:

Withdrawal potential. A person with severe dependence on alcohol with a history of withdrawal complications or withdrawal seizures would be recommended for medically supervised detoxification in a hospital setting before other treatment services are used.

Biomedical conditions and complications. A person with a history of seizures or concurrent diabetes would be recommended for treatment in a setting in which medical care is available.

Emotional conditions or complications. If the person with the AUD has a psychiatric disorder of such severity to require psychiatric management or medications, treatment in a "dual diagnosis" program in a psychiatric system would be preferred over treatment in a substance abuse clinic.

Treatment acceptance. The motivation of the person with the AUD often determines whether treatment recommendations are accepted or followed. For example, a professional may recommend a residential rehabilitation program due to the severity of the addiction, but the person with the AUD may refuse the recommendation. This refusal may result from low motivation to change, failure to accept the severity of the AUD, or resistance to taking time off work to attend a treatment program.

Recovery environment and social support. The availability of supportive family, friends or community groups plays a role in treatment recommendations. Some environments are more conducive to recovery than others. For example, if a person dependent on alcohol lives with family members or friends who drink excessively, a residential program may be recommended in order to help this person evaluate whether it is in the person's best interest to return to such an environment upon completing the program.

Relapse potential. The person's history of problems with the AUD, prior attempts at treatment and recovery, and history of relapses impact on treatment decisions. For example, a person with an extensive history of failing to stay sober despite participation in a variety of treatment programs may be encouraged to use a medication to assist in staying sober.

(continued on page 78)

The Whites of His Eyes
Leslie Smith Townsend

I noticed the whites of his eyes on a blustery gray November day in 2000. Sarah, my twelve-year-old daughter and I had gone to my parents' house to rake leaves. My brother Bruce stood in front of the open garage at the base of the steeply sloped drive, eyes glazed, leaf blower dangling in his left hand. His features—baby blue eyes, ski jump nose, and classic jaw *(Oh, he'd once been so handsome)*—were lost amid folds of puffy flesh, making him appear older than his forty-nine years. He wore a baseball cap, t-shirt stained brown with old blood and dirty blue jeans. Dried blood matted his sandy beard. Mom said he'd been having nosebleeds.

"Hi, Bruce," I said as I walked down the driveway.

"Hi," Sarah echoed.

Bruce lifted his head slowly and regarded us. He seemed far away, as if submerged in fathoms of water, struggling to break free of the depths that held him. "Hi," he said.

His hands shook with tremors. With great effort, he lifted the leaf blower, brought his right hand around to the pull cord, and attempted to yank it. It didn't budge. Bruce stared at the lifeless object in his hands, as if not comprehending. Sarah and I watched mutely as he tried again. "Damn cord," Bruce muttered as his right hand flailed spastically.

"Here, Bruce. Let me have a try," Sarah offered.

I watched skeptically. Sarah was small for her age, still under five feet and weighing eighty-two pounds. She whipped her long brown hair over one shoulder and yanked the cord. The blower sputtered and sparked and vibrated in her hands. Bruce's head bobbed in silent acknowledgement as he watched Sarah blow crackly, brown oak leaves into a pile along the driveway.

Gazing at Sarah, I thought of when I was twelve and Bruce was fourteen, and we'd just moved into this house perched on a cliff with woods and a winding brook below and towers of creek rock that we used as fortresses for our adventures. We'd fashion bows and arrows from fallen branches and send them soaring and flaming (so we imagined) down the hillside to penetrate the hearts of our enemies. Bruce skirted the cliffs in the Keene's backyard while I covered him from behind a mossy boulder that smelled of rich humus and new beginnings. "Hey Leslie," he hollered. "Come here quick." I darted along the cliff line till I joined him. "It's a cave, see? It's got an opening on two sides."

Bruce tapped me on the arm and interrupted my reverie. "Tell her to blow the leaves onto the plastic."

"Okay."

I directed Sarah toward a large plastic sheet spread across the center of the lawn. She quickly filled the sheet full of leaves and turned off the blower. Bruce moved unevenly across the grass and picked up one corner of the plastic. Sarah and I each grabbed a corner and began carrying the load around the side of the house toward the backyard. Bruce stumbled and let go.

"We can manage," I said. "You take a break." Bruce watched us for a moment, then turned and staggered uphill to the front yard.

The back yard dropped off abruptly along the edge of a cliff. Sarah and I dragged the plastic across the grass, counted to three, then hoisted the leaves over the bluff, watching as they tumbled onto moss-covered rocks and Virginia creeper. "Good job," I said. "You've got muscle on those bones."

Sarah smiled and took my hand as we walked around the house to the front yard, pulling the sheet of plastic behind us.

"Hey Sarah, you come to help, too?" Mom called from the front porch.

"Hi Mimi, got any candy for me?"

"Guess you'll have to come inside after you're done and find out."

Mom stood on the front porch watching as Sarah steered the leaf blower and I raked. Bruce nudged me. "Get the pile at the top of the hill." He pointed and Sarah followed, scattering leaves in the air like dustbowls on the prairie. "Aim that thing closer to the ground," Bruce said.

Sarah and I carried two more loads of leaves around the back, making a game of tossing them over the cliff, seeing how far we could fling them, watching them dance and twirl and spin in the damp air. "I'm tired, Mom," she said. "Can I go inside for awhile?"

"Sure, Sweetie. I'll finish up."

I finished raking and walked into the house to get Sarah. She grabbed her sweatshirt and candy, called good-bye to Mimi, and climbed the hill to the car.

"Come on, Mom," she hollered, leaning out of the passenger-side door. "You wanted to go, so let's go."

Bruce stopped me in the green dip of yard along the stepping stones. We stood face to face. He told me that he and Mom had had a fight—that Mom told him he couldn't hang around all the time. He had to go home by six o'clock at night.

I looked into his eyes. The whites were lemon yellow. I remember thinking: my brother is dying.

Two weeks later, on Thanksgiving morning, I called Bruce. He picked up the phone after seven or eight rings. "Hey Bruce, I wanted to make sure you knew about Thanksgiving dinner. We're going to eat around 4:30."

"I'm not coming."

"Why not?"

"I've been having trouble. I've got all this dried blood in my mustache. Do you know anything that would get it out?"

"You might try a warm washcloth. Lay it across your face. If you fill a bowl with hot water, you won't have to get up as often."

"Yeah, I think I'll try that. I'm okay when I lay down, but if I stand or sit up, my nose starts bleeding."

"Do you have a recliner?"

"Yeah. That old one Dad got me from Sears. It doesn't work well anymore."

"When you stand up, do you get dizzy?"

"Not really, but I feel kind of lightheaded. I've been bumping into things. That's why I want to stay home. I know where everything is."

"Bruce, do you want me to take you to the doctor?"

"No. I'm okay. It's just sinus stuff. The heat keeps coming on and drying me out."

I pleaded with him to let me take him to the hospital, knowing that he wouldn't. A year earlier, Bruce had suffered two alcohol-related seizures while on vacation with my parents. Since that time, they'd bribed and threatened, but Bruce refused to see a doctor. He must have feared he'd lose the two freedoms most precious to him: drinking and driving. Finally, I signed off, "If you need anything, give me a call."

You might think I wrestled with the decision to leave my brother alone. Instead, I hung up the phone and returned to Thanksgiving dinner preparations. Perhaps my husband, Loren, and I should have loaded the dead weight of Bruce's inebriated body into the passenger seat of my Toyota and carted him to the hospital.

I played out the scenario in my mind—Bruce detoxed of booze and discharged from the hospital to his one room apartment and jobless life. How long till he picked up the bottle? One day? One week? I couldn't imagine him attending A.A. Bruce had never admitted he had a problem in his life. Everything was someone else's fault.

The simple truth was that I couldn't put into action a plan I couldn't envision. I couldn't picture Bruce apart from his booze, isolation, and angry defiance. More than that, I was swept up in a family ethos that dictated we not interfere—that if nothing else, we should preserve each other's autonomy. It's not healthy detachment I'm speaking of here, the kind you learn at Al-Anon meetings. No, I'd learned not to notice when Bruce slipped from boisterous to tipsy, teenage drinking to alcoholism, athletic discipline to stumbling over the dog and passing out cold. I had learned to look the other way.

As I checked the meat thermometer on the turkey, an image of Bruce lying in a rickety recliner with blood oozing down his chin and onto his shirt seized me. This image slid out of focus and another emerged: Bruce lying on a hardwood floor in a pool of blood, dead.

"I told him to put Vaseline under his nose," Mom said, taking a sip of her Screwdriver. She lifted the lid off the potatoes boiling on my stove. The scent of garden-rich loam mixed with sage and roasting turkey. Minutes later, Mom realized she'd forgotten the onion water for the gravy. "I'll call Bruce and have him run it over."

Bruce lived down the street from me in a vinyl-sided two-story duplex that Mom and Dad owned. "Running it over" meant he'd climb in his car, drive five miles to our parent's house, and five miles back. "Mom, he's dying!" I wanted to scream, but instead, said, "Forget it, Mom. The gravy will be fine."

When the turkey finished roasting, we gathered around the table. Loren and I had been married a little over one year. His children, Nathan and Leslea, twenty-two and twenty-one, joined my girls, Chelsea and Sarah, who were fifteen and twelve. Dad, who suffered from Parkinson's disease, shuffled to his seat as I pulled out his chair. Mom placed dinner rolls on the table and took a seat next to Dad. Everyone paused while I offered thanks, "Bless this food to our use and us to thy loving service. Keep us ever mindful of the needs of others. Amen."

As I passed broccoli casserole and sweet potatoes, I thought of Bruce down the street. How odd it seemed to celebrate Thanksgiving as if nothing were amiss. Should I say something?

I glanced at my mother sitting catty-cornered to me at the dining room table. She speared a piece of broccoli and raised it to her mouth. Her cool composure stopped me. Any expression of concern would challenge her detachment—her denial that Bruce suffered anything more than a cold.

After dinner, I served decaf coffee and pecan pie. Loren and Dad watched football while Mom and I cleaned up and divided leftovers.

Less than a block away, Bruce sopped up blood with a warm washcloth.

As teenagers, both Bruce and I drank, with the only difference being that I fell asleep and woke up puking. Eventually, I tired of the ritual—the waiting, my head over a commode with gut searing nausea and the smell of boozy phlegm rising, till I retched again and again. Bruce was formed from stronger stuff. As he kicked back Budweisers with buddies playing pool—so sleek, his muscles taut, his swagger poised and confident—I imagined liquor stirring in him a sense of power, the fulfillment of his lifelong dream: the dream of being "normal." And he needed normalcy. When Bruce was six years old, he had been diagnosed as severely emotionally disturbed. Less than a year later, he became the first child in Kentucky to be diagnosed as perceptually handicapped— a term that is no longer used. Today, Bruce's problems would be labeled learning disabilities with Attention Deficit Disorder, hyperactive type.

I defined my life in juxtaposition to my struggling brother. When he failed, I cursed myself. When he accused, I defended, while secretly harboring the same conclusions he'd come to: Life wasn't fair; I'd wrested the winning hand from his grasping fingers. My ground was shaped with the same compulsion as Bruce's, the same longing to escape, the same craving for self-obliteration.

Something happened in the weeks my brother lay dying. For the first time since we were preschoolers, Bruce let me love him, and he loved me back.

Bruce drifted to sleep on a gurney in the emergency room. I sat down on a cold, vinyl chair and tried to read, but I couldn't concentrate. My mind wandered back to the day before when I'd made a last-ditch attempt to get Bruce to a doctor.

"You need to sign these forms, Bruce," I'd said, thrusting several pages at him as he rested in his recliner.

"Why?" he'd asked.

"You need to see a doctor."

"Leave them on the table," he'd said. "I'll look at them later."

I set my book down and gazed at Bruce. His skin was the color of spicy mustard. His bloated belly rose and fell in rhythm with his breathing. What would happen to him here, and what did Bruce think of submitting to medical treatment after resisting for so long? He wouldn't be here now except my parent's neighbor, a nurse, had convinced my mother that Bruce would soon be dead if she didn't take him to the hospital. Had he argued with Mom when she told him to get into the car?

My thoughts were interrupted by a physician with a steel-gray medical chart in his hands. He motioned me into the hallway where he introduced himself as Dr. Jones. After asking me several questions, he approached Bruce.

"Bruce, wake up. Can you hear me? Wake up."

Bruce opened his eyes and looked at the doctor looming over him.

"When you were at home, how much alcohol did you drink each day?"

Surely he doesn't expect an accurate answer.

Bruce glanced at me and back at Dr. Jones. "Maybe two or three beers a night."

"How long have you been drinking?"

I did the math. *He's forty-nine now and started drinking at fifteen. That makes thirty-four years.*

Bruce squinted in concentration. "A while, I guess."

Dr. Jones crossed his arms over his chest and straightened up so that only his head tipped toward Bruce. "Now listen to me, Bruce." His voice deepened and swelled. "You're an alcoholic. Drinking has poisoned your liver. You are very, very sick."

Bruce nodded his head and looked straight into the doctor's eyes.

"You have to stop drinking. You have no choice. If you drink again, you will die. Do you understand me?"

"Yes, sir," Bruce nodded. "I understand. I won't drink anymore."

"Good."

I followed Dr. Jones out of the room. "What's his prognosis?" I asked.

"It depends on the extent of damage to the liver. If it's not too bad, the liver can repair itself. We'll have to wait and see."

Bruce died six weeks later. Though he never said, "I love you, Leslie," I take comfort in the fact that he trusted me. And how could he trust me if he didn't first love me?

Leslie Smith Townsend holds a PhD from Southern Baptist Theological Seminary and an MFA from Spalding University. She has published many professional articles and book reviews in the fields of theology, pastoral care, spirituality, and death and dying. Her story is an excerpt from her memoir, *Body Beautiful: A Memoir of Alcoholism*. Townsend is a recipient of a Studio Saturday award from the Indiana Arts Commission (2004) and the Betty Gabehart prize in Creative Nonfiction from the Kentucky Women's Writers Conference (2005). Her work has been published in *The New Southerner*, *The Louisville Review*, *Arable*, and *Church and Society*. When she's not writing, Townsend works as a licensed marriage and family therapist in private practice.

Family Tree
Katrina Cleveland

Mom met Richard when I was seven or eight years old, I don't remember exactly. I loved him at first, and thought the world of him. My own dad lived a thousand miles away and I never got to see him. Later that year, she married him and he became my stepdad. I was cool with this arrangement; at first, he was a really great guy. In the end, he was still a good guy. But when he drank, he was the meanest man I have ever known. Mom knew Richard was an alcoholic, but I guess she was just a poor judge of men and she married him anyway. I dubbed him "The Alkie."

It started getting bad when I was ten and we moved to Grantsville, Utah. I was happy there, at first. I was in the fourth grade and ready for a fresh start. We could have a horse and a good life, I thought. I was always optimistic. But when the days got short and the nights got long, my stepdad started coming home from work drunk. He used our rent money to buy vodka. From time to time, he used the phone money and we had no phone. Sometimes he used the gas money and we had no heat. He used the food money and we were thankful for school lunches. One night, he stole my sister's babysitting money; she was twelve years old and saving up for her horse. She had saved $300: he took it all. But the stealing wasn't the hard part, it turned out. The hard part was the violence.

Mom and Richard got in a fight one night, a bad one. My mom was 5 foot 9 and weighed 110 pounds. Richard was 6 foot 3 and outweighed her by at least 140 pounds but the vodka evened things out. I listened as their argument echoed through our tiny house. They were beating on each other and screaming like banshees. I didn't know what to do; I was hiding, more like cowering, if truth be known, in the bedroom I shared with my sister. I heard their bedroom door slam shut. Then I heard a thud and then, silence. I was scared. No more hollering, just silence. I took the two steps from my bedroom to theirs, put my hand on their door and pushed it hard.

My mom was sprawled on the bed, her head in his lap, not three feet from where I stood. Richard was choking her. Her eyes were rolled into the back of her head so only the whites showed. Her face was whiter than snow, her lips were blue. I thought she was dead; I knew she was dead, she had to be. I screamed at him and he let her go. He was shocked at what he had done. I ran back into my room and crawled out the window and ran to the barn. I do not remember coming back to the house, though I assume I did. Mom didn't die that night.

Soon after, there was another big fight. It died out quickly, and Richard passed out in bed. But Mom had had enough. She locked herself in the bathroom and then fell into the bathtub full of old bath water. My mom was sick of living, I suppose, and my sister and I watched her through the keyhole as she grabbed the pill box, watched as the pills went into her mouth.

My sister screamed at me to call the police. I called, then ran out to the end of the gravel driveway to wait for them. I was crying when they arrived. I tried to run with them into the house; I made it there as they broke down the door. I saw my mom in her white coat, her eyes red and swollen. They lifted her out and put her on a stretcher and into the ambulance. My stepdad slept through the whole thing. Mom was released from the hospital two days later.

When I was 12, while I sat in our Bronco with Mom, she told me that I would either be an alcoholic or I would marry an alcoholic and repeat the cycle. That was not something I wanted to hear when I was 12. But I was terrified, and I made sure it wasn't going to happen to me. Today, I am married to a good man who never drinks and never will. In fact, I married a cop. Talk about irony. But I never forgot what my mom said to me that day about the cycle of alcoholism and I decided I wouldn't live that life, like my mom did and her mom before her. Alcoholism in my family stops with me.

Katrina Cleveland is the 24-year-old mother of two-year-old Anikah with another on the way.

(continued from page 64)

What Motivates People with AUDs to Get Help?

...I began my night with wine-in-a-box and pizza bites. I was having a pity party over a recent breakup... I devised a plan to drive to Cannery Row in disguise and hunt down my ex.... Before my saturated forebrain could calculate my next move, we were tag-teamed by two officers.... A limo driver had called in a citizen's arrest after he watched me park.... I am now in an 18-month multiple offender program... two hours a week, twelve of us meet for "group"... and six mandatory education classes... there's also a 15-minute "face to "face' with the group counselor... my home confinement program will last for 39 days....This experience has finally gotten me on the right path....
—Lisa, *To Drink or Not to Drink*, page 123

...It took four more DWI's, a near-divorce and more than fourteen month's total prison time before my eyes finally opened. I missed Christmas and Thanksgiving dinners. I missed a whole lot of important things I took for granted anyway... I hid my drinking from my wife for about four months, then I drank openly in front of her. It was like a slap in the face to her; and that's when she began to fall out of love with me... I couldn't live like this any longer... I immersed myself in recovery... I gave my addictions over to God and my cries for help were answered because I was ready to help myself...
—Steven, *The Path was Rocky (But Worth It)*, page 97

> ...*For many of us alcoholics, especially those "high bottom drunks" like me who haven't lost everything yet, reaching the point of facing reality doesn't arrive quickly ... we continue to function for years and years, gradually acknowledging to ourselves that we have a problem with alcohol but are too ashamed, too powerless, too ignorant to do anything about it.... I was able to observe my withdrawal from my grandchildren, my relationships with my children and my friendships, not to mention my marriage. It wasn't until years later that I saw clearly the utter selfishness of my life as it deteriorated...*
> —Karen, *The Healing Power of Truth*, page 51

As the stories in this book show, people with AUDs get help for many reasons. Some, like Karen, realize their drinking is affecting their life or family and decide to take action. Others, like Lisa, give in to pressure from the legal system or an employer and get help. Still others, like Steven, decide to get help following a dose of reality from loved ones.

Individuals with AUDs often deny that their drinking is a problem or refuse to acknowledge the negative effects of these problems on their lives or the lives of family members. As a result, they may believe they do not need treatment. They may believe that they can change on their own without the help of others. Motivational strategies may be used to increase a person's readiness for treatment and motivation to change. External pressure from the legal system, an employer, or the family is often the reason a person with alcoholism initially gets help.

There is a saying that "you can lead a horse to water but not make him drink it." But you can make him thirsty. In other words, anyone who influences a reluctant alcoholic to enter treatment exposes this person to a program that can make him or her "thirsty" for sobriety.

It is not unusual for motivation to be external at first, and then become internalized after the person spends time in a treatment program.

(continued on page 91)

I Really Am Special
Julie Anne Hunter

While many people sit back and fondly recall the memories of their childhoods, I do everything possible to forget mine. While I'm sure there had to be some very special times, most of the joy was clouded by living with my father. He was a very sick, selfish man who made life hell for all of us. But the ugliest side of Dad, the one I saw most often, was caused by his alcoholism.

While my classmates would count the days until Christmas, I prayed my family would somehow make it through another major uproar, since holiday parties always included alcohol. Back then, it was common to keep such troubles quiet. You went to school and acted normal. You went to Sunday mass as a family, carrying all the sadness and fear inside. We were so good at this deception that people called us the "model" family. Little did they know that our family was falling apart.

Although my mother bore the brunt of my father's rage, my sister and I were never far from it. I still shake today, thinking back to the nights when we lay in our beds and listened while Dad used Mom for a punching bag. He would rant and call her profane names. We'd hear Mom's screams as she hit the floor. He beat her, once so badly she miscarried. We were instructed not to tell anyone.

My mother worked nights. After she left for work, Dad would make my brother and me go to bed so he could spend the night alone with my sister. She was a high school senior at the time and I was a naïve little freshman. I knew that my dad adored her, and I always wondered why I meant nothing to him. Since it was summer and we didn't have to get up for school, we complained to Mom about the early bedtime. When Dad found out that we told on him, he was furious. He beat us and told us to keep our mouths shut. After that, we did.

One night I was home alone with Dad. He was drunk. He told me he loved me and asked me to come and sit on the floor in front of him. This spot usually belonged to my sister. I was elated! My father finally wanted to be close to me. But before I knew it, his hands began to wander to my chest. My heart was screaming for help. I had never before gone against my father's wishes, but at that moment, I really didn't care if he got mad and killed me. Almost reflexively I brought my knee up and hit him between his legs. He screamed in pain; I jumped up, ran to my bedroom and slammed the door. But he was right on my heels. Dad burst into the room and made me promise not to tell anyone what he had done, telling me if I told on him they'd put him in jail. Then he left me alone to cry.

What had I done to deserve this? I sat on the floor next to the open window and wept my heart out. Mom would still be gone for six more hours. How would I survive?

That night, my father made hourly visits to my room. He wanted my assurance that I would not tell on him. Out of fear for my life, I agreed to keep "our secret." But I knew I would tell Mom the first chance I could. I didn't care if he went to jail. I didn't wish him dead, but I prayed that he could just disappear forever.

Morning came. Dad went to work, and Mom came home and went to bed. I got up and started crying louder and louder. I wanted her to hear me. She did. She asked me what was wrong, and I told her. She locked me away in my aunt's house for a week, until she could quit work and stay home with us. I found out during that time that my father had been sleeping with my sister for several years. He had threatened her life, and she was too scared to tell anyone.

Time passed, and my parents stayed together. My sister went to college, and the fighting seemed to subside a little. My father hated me for telling on him, and he told me every chance he got that I was *worthless* and would *never amount to anything*. I started to believe it. I had low self-esteem, and became a loner. Why would anyone even want to be with me? By then my biggest goal was to move away from my father. I dated a guy and hoped we would get married so I could move away, but he turned out to be unfaithful and it broke my heart.

Then I met my husband. It took everything he had to prove to me that "not all men are created equal." With endless persuasion and gentleness he convinced me to marry him.

We had five kids in six years. I often thought back to my dad telling me I would never amount to anything. But I knew I was a good wife and mother. My life seemed almost *too perfect*. That near perfection didn't last long. I was diagnosed with multiple sclerosis. I had seen people with MS; I thought I would become a burden to my family. I was so distraught I told my husband I wanted a divorce, to free him from the burden of caring for me. But he dismissed my fears, told me he loved me and that we were in it together. His words meant so much.

The day following my diagnosis, my father told me, for the first time ever, that he loved me. I knew the love he was speaking of was a beautiful, clean and tender love. He never told me again, but once was enough.

My dad continued to drink to excess. I didn't hate him, nor did I like him; I built a wall between him and my emotions where I felt safe. Eventually, my mother and father were diagnosed with Alzheimer's disease at virtually the same time. The doctors told us that Dad's condition was brought on by his alcoholism. They both ended up in the same nursing home. I watched my father as he withdrew from the alcohol, and understood how scary that experience is for someone like him.

A short time later he had a stroke, leaving him paralyzed from the neck down. He also developed an incurable staph infection. Seeing him in this state, my emotions changed again. I went to the nursing home weekly to visit my parents. My father was no longer this giant monster waiting to lunge at me; I was no longer afraid of him. He was just one of the many elderly there, in terrible pain. He was lonely and looking for even the least bit of love.

Mom passed away but I continued to see my father. Because of the staph infection, my doctors warned me not to touch him. But here was a man with no other visitors, with eyes begging for someone, anyone, to care about him. I knew I had to do what both Mom and God would want me to do. I gambled with fate and held my father's hands and squeezed them so he knew that someone was there for him.

One morning I got a call from the nursing home. Dad was dying. I had never seen anyone die, and I was not sure I could deal with it. For three hours I sat at his side, holding his hands, the same hands that so many years before had abused me. I used cotton swabs dipped in water to moisten his lips to make him more comfortable, the same lips that had told me so often I would never amount to anything.

In the afternoon, Dad opened his eyes. He looked straight at me. I said, "I'm here, Daddy, it's okay, Mom is waiting for you." Dad smiled at me, closed his eyes and took his last breath.

I believe that if Dad had found some help, all of our lives might have turned out differently. I know we can't go back. I am so glad to live in a time when you can admit you are an alcoholic and there are many great people to support you. I can't change my past, but I live to be a positive part of the future for others. I want to be that someone who helps, because you see, my father was wrong. I *am* someone special.

Julie Anne Hunter is the pseudonym of this prolific writer who has had published eleven stories in the *Chicken Soup for the Soul* books series, three children books, and articles in over 40 national and international magazines.

Mothers Can't Be Drunks, Can They?
Valerie Scully

When you're young, your parents are your entire world. They are the first people you meet and your first exposure to life. They are your teachers, your cheerleaders, your providers, your friends, your teammates. They are perfect people who can do no wrong. Parents are your "everything" during childhood.

My rosy view changed when I turned sixteen and my stepfather and I took my mother to rehab for alcoholism. It was an unreal situation for me: she was my mother and, therefore, she had to be perfect. I thought it was normal for her to drink wine at 9:00 A.M. and that there was nothing odd in finding half-full glasses of wine in the kitchen cabinets. Isn't "Bloody Mary" part of the vocabulary of every five-year-old? Doesn't every family have boxes of wine stashed in the basement?

My stepfather had gone through rehabilitation for alcoholism himself about ten years earlier. I was young then, and I don't remember much from that time. But he still attended Alcoholics Anonymous, so I was a bit familiar with the recovery process and what rehab would be like for my mother. I knew I'd be able to visit her, and that I would have to go to those silly family sessions.

We left Mom at detox and went home. I was actually a bit happy: I was excited to be able to use her car while she was away. I was deeply involved with my boyfriend at the time and, like most sixteen-year-olds, I was focused primarily on myself. I remember thinking that Mom probably wouldn't be in there long since she really wasn't that much of an alcoholic: I just wasn't able to think negatively about my mother. When I imagined an alcoholic, the image of a dirty bum on the curb of a city street with a wine bottle wrapped in a paper bag in hand came to mind. That was not my mother. She was a nice, well-liked Christian woman. She didn't go out to bars every night, nor did she scream and holler in drunken rages when she had a bad day. To me, she just liked to have a few drinks. What could be wrong with that?

I don't remember a lot about the time she was in rehab, which lasted about a month. I went to see her there with my boyfriend, who seemed to be more concerned about my mother's mental and physical state than I was. But I was in denial at that time: I wanted to believe Mom was just a bit stressed out and needed a break for a bit.

The months after she returned home from rehab were not fun. My mother and stepfather's marriage nearly ended. I struggled with accepting that my mother really was an alcoholic, and all of us went to A.A. meetings. Because I did not want to be at home to deal with my family, I buried myself more and more deeply in my relationship with my boyfriend. Surprisingly, my schoolwork didn't suffer, and I was still on track for college. I am very grateful for that; I imagine others in the same position would have had a difficult time dealing with school or work.

I finally realized, during the year after my mother came home, that she was a vulnerable, recovering addict. I finally understood that she was not just my mother, but a person, one who needed help and would continue to need help. I also got over feeling obligated to take care of her. I knew that she needed to learn how to take care of herself.

But still, I struggled. I hated life at home. My mom and my stepfather fought constantly; I guess a seasoned, recovering alcoholic and a newly recovering alcoholic don't mix well. I was starting to apply to colleges and became concerned about leaving my mother. If my mother and stepfather's marriage failed, who would take care of her? If I weren't there, would she be okay?

I did not handle any of this well. I became self-destructive, both physically and emotionally. I thought about killing myself, but what I wanted was to get rid of the hurt, the negative feelings and the constant tension. I was sent to a mental facility myself for a month during my senior year of high school. My mother was away on business and my father unreachable when I admitted to my school guidance counselor that I needed help. I ended up being driven to a mental facility by two police officers. It was an experience I never want to relive.

My recovery involved a lot of discussion about my mother and my real father. I attended Children of Alcoholics sessions and really dove into my feelings and experiences. It was not a fun period, but it helped me deal with everything that had happened in my life. I finally admitted that my mother was indeed an alcoholic and would always be one. I finally realized that I didn't have to be perfect, something I didn't believe at the time; I felt I had to be responsible at all times, that messing up was not allowed. I struggle with guilt to this day.

Today, I thank God that we all made it through. My mother and my stepfather are still married and attending A.A. I graduated college and I am happy with my life. The tools I learned during my stay in the mental hospital and from A.A., Children of Alcoholics and Al-Anon have helped me tremendously. I am thankful that programs such as these exist.

To others who might be going through times like these, or those who feel they have nowhere to turn, never give up. There are organizations and people out there who really do care about you.

Life is not easy, but it is really worth living. I've been through enough to know that every day is a gift. First we have to accept it, and then use it and enjoy it the best we can.

A graduate of William and Mary College, the author currently lives in Dallas, Texas. She has spent the past eight years as a technical writer and is currently working on a collection of humor essays.

(continued from page 80)

What Treatments Are Available for AUD's?

The majority of individuals with AUDs never receive medical treatment. But, while some are able to stop using on their own or with the help of mutual support programs such as Alcoholics Anonymous (A.A.), others require professional treatment to help them stop using alcohol and to make changes in themselves and their lifestyle in order to remain sober.

The person with an AUD may enter treatment voluntarily or involuntarily as a result of any of the following: personally realizing that alcohol use is a problem and help is needed to deal with it and the other problems it causes; taking the advice of a concerned person or loved one; giving in to pressure from a formal "intervention" in which loved ones meet together with the person with the AUD and present their view of the situation and share observations of the person's substance use, impaired behaviors, and how they have been affected; or a legal mandate by a court imposed as a result of a charge or conviction of a crime in which alcohol use was a factor, such as driving under the influence of alcohol.

Treatment of AUDs requires a range of services that can meet the needs of people with different types and severity of AUDs. It includes professional services specific for AUDs, services for other types of problems (e.g., medical or psychiatric), and mutual support programs such as A.A.

The American Society on Addiction Medicine recommends that treatment be "matched" to the problems of the individual with the AUD. Treatment settings from the least to the most intensive include the following:

Outpatient counseling (OPT). Individual, group and/or family counseling may be offered. Frequency of sessions depends on the needs and problems of the individual with the AUD and/or the concerns of the family. Many start with weekly sessions and then taper off as treatment progresses. Individual counseling involves talking one-on-one with an addiction medicine professional, usually for up to an hour at a time. Group counseling involves meeting with one or two counselors with a group of other individuals, usually for up to two hours at a time. The goals of OPT may be to determine if an AUD exists and what to do about it; stopping substance use; making personal changes to support abstinence; learning to spot early signs of relapse; and dealing with problems contributing to or resulting from the AUD.

Intensive Outpatient (IOP) or Partial Hospital (PH) programs. IOP and PH programs have the same goals: to help the person become sober and learn skills to stay sober over time. Individual, family and group counseling may be offered as part of IOP or PH programs. IOP is less intensive than PH, and may involve the person attending a program 3 to5 days a week, for up to 10 hours of education and counseling. A PH program usually involves attending sessions 5 to 7 days a week for up to 20 hours or more a week, for two to six weeks.

Ambulatory detoxification. Some addiction medicine clinics offer *supervised detoxification* in addition to OPT, IOP or PH services. This service involves meeting with a health care professional, usually a nurse and doctor, who monitors the person's withdrawal symptoms and vital signs. Counseling and education are often provided as part of the sessions with the nurse or physician. Medications may be ordered one day at a time to help the person safely withdraw from alcohol or other drugs. This service usually lasts just a few days, and its goal is to get the person being detoxified to remain in treatment. If withdrawal symptoms worsen significantly, the person may be referred to an inpatient detoxification unit in a hospital or rehabilitation program.

Residential rehabilitation programs. A primary rehabilitation program lasts up to three or four weeks; a halfway house program (HWH) lasts several months or longer. Both aim to provide education, support and counseling to help the person with the AUD learn how to stay sober and solve problems without relapsing to alcohol use. Many programs use addiction counselors who have personal experiences with recovery from alcoholism. A primary rehabilitation program provides a structured treatment day in which the person attends many different types of programs, including recovery education groups, therapy groups, individual counseling, leisure or recreational counseling, and mutual support groups such as AA. Clients are often asked to write an extensive history of alcohol and drug use and then share this with a counseling group. Peers can then share their opinions on the seriousness of the person's AUD.

Medical detoxification. This occurs on a medically managed unit in a hospital or a medically monitored unit of a rehabilitation program. Medical detoxification is for individuals with more severe withdrawal syndromes or those with significant medical problems in addition to an active addiction. Detoxification usually lasts 2 to 5 days and involves monitoring withdrawal symptoms, taking medications if symptoms warrant this, and participating in educational or counseling services.

While some individuals use only one type of service discussed, others use multiple services, either during the course of their current episode or as a result of relapses following periods of sobriety. Those who's AUDs include dependence often have a chronic form of addiction. Like chronic medical or psychiatric disorders, their alcoholism may require recurrent treatment over time.

(continued on page 112)

The Day He Left
Allison S. Jones

Trying to control Brian's drinking made me insane. I was no longer able to separate the disease from the man. So I gave him a week to pack up his things and leave. I felt courageous, empowered and scared. What was I doing? I had two small boys, how would I survive?

Even though he had been in a program for a year, Brian was struggling. His sulky demeanor and uneven temper made me realize that, while he might be attending A.A. meetings, he was drowning in himself. Brian didn't believe me when I told him he needed to leave. I explained as calmly as I could that his behavior was unacceptable and that we needed to be apart. His eyes were empty: no pride; plenty of pain.

The day he was to leave, I arranged to have the boys and myself out of the house. He left with one garbage bag filled with his possessions to his new home: he would now live next door to some drug dealers, across the street from a strip club. I knew this was the right decision for our family; a step towards healing from the effects of the disease. However, I knew that it was going to be difficult for the boys, then aged seven and three, to understand. I could only try to make them feel secure and loved. Everything else was out of my power. When we returned to the empty house, the silence was suffocating. The sadness was overwhelming. How did we get here?

It wasn't a case of not loving Brian. But I loved myself enough to ask for what I needed, and I needed him to leave. I could no longer worry about his disease and how he was working the program. In the short time that I myself had been in Al Anon, I'd learned that I didn't cause his disease, I couldn't control it, and I couldn't cure it. What I could do was take care of myself and my children and pray that Brian would find his way back to us.

My mom thought I was nuts. "Why are you kicking out the father of your children?" she asked. "Don't you remember your vows?" I had hoped she would understand and be supportive, but she was afraid that her daughter would become a single mother. I was afraid of that too. The separation seemed like years. We worked diligently on our respective programs, hoping that by loving and improving ourselves we could become a better unit.

One morning, the phone rang at 4:30 A.M. I heard the hysterical voice of my mother, begging me to call Brian and get over to her house right away. My father had taken ill and needed to be taken to the hospital. Brian and I met at the house. We got Dad to the hospital; his condition was critical and it would eventually cost him his leg. During Dad's recovery, Brian was there for me. With his steady support and unconditional love, Brian gave me a gift that in years past would have been impossible.

Two months after we had separated, Brian came home to stay. Our relationship has since come a long way. We still struggle, but today we have our recovery programs and strong sponsors who help us faithfully. The effects of alcoholism will be forever with us, but today active alcoholism is not a factor.

There are no victims in this disease, only willing participants. My part was trying to change and control something over which I was completely powerless. But allowing myself to see that there are no victims, I was able to forgive myself and Brian. The transformation is slow and I grow each day in the knowledge that I am an eager student with much to learn.

Allison S. Jones is a freelance writer who resides in Louisville, Kentucky with her husband, Brian, and her sons Bailey and Bryce. She received a master's degree in writing from Spalding University.

Guilty Feet Have Got No Rhythm
Angela Lovell

She wakes and pulls the green oxygen tube out of her nose to scratch a tiny itch, her features porcelain even in this lighting. She resembles a gifted child in her delicacy to reinsert it. Noticing me next to her hospital bed, she mumbles, "Are you bored?"

"Not at all."

"I'm sorry about all this."

"Don't be. I love you."

"I love you more."

I am not gay, but I realize as I rush back to the hospital that I am madly in love with a girl. A girl whose bed I share, a girl who flosses as I sit on the toilet, a girl whose underwear and Monopoly game I packed into a busting red suitcase and toted all the way to the East Village, a girl whose absence from my life would leave me much more pitiful and weakened than would the absence of any man. A girl whose drinking is a problem.

"Angie, it wasn't even a good song! If it had been 'Welcome to the Jungle' it would have been justified!"

I first find Ruby lying in bed 12 at Beth Israel's emergency room. She has been alone all night, which hurts me with the appearance of an unfamiliar intruder—Guilt. Fourteen times Thursday night she called my cell phone, screaming, crying, terrified, threatening, and assuming I ignored her constant rings, as though such a thing is possible. Calling too many late nights, ruining my 9-to-5-er sleep schedule, training me to turn my ringer off before bed, Ruby was the girl who cried wolf. Thursday night I was exhausted but inspired by a great script meeting and just wanted to get my Zen on in my new sublet. Ruby was downtown and on the go, as always. She headed to an eastside dive where our non-fictitious character, by the name "Faggy Elf," tends bar. Rube finds him attractive. I find him faggy.

Faggy Elf was being wooed by other alpha females that night. Ruby was working hard to catch his eye, despite all the free tequila shots he'd been dousing her with. She was working so hard that she climbed onto the bar in 4½" platforms and proceeded to dance next to the girl who was winning Faggy Elf's affections. How Rube managed to get onto the bar, we do not know. The fall, however, was inevitable. Landing behind the bar, taking bottles of booze with her, Ruby lay for a moment assessing the damage to her body. Faggy Elf quickly approached, flailing like a gangly school teacher, "Are you alright?!"

Ruby told the nervous elf she was not all right, but moments later a bouncer was yanking her arm and pulling her out from behind the bar. Ruby hobbled to a couch in back, handing her cell phone to a stranger and asking him, "Please call me an ambulance... But don't tell anybody."

The three EMTs who locked and loaded my battered friend were all women.

"Ma'am, are you intoxicated?"

"What do you think? I was dancing on a bar!"

At 3 A.M. on Friday morning, Ruby is left in the ER. I do not reach her until 10 A.M. after I unlock my office for friendly capitalists. I do not know how I got from A to B doing what had to be done, knowing she needed me, but I did. I cannot afford to lose this job.

She has not slept. She sobbed all night. She's had no food since noon the day before. But when I find my best friend in bed 12 she is happy, wearing a hospital gown, pantiless, glad to see me, and mostly just jacked up on morphine and still rather drunk. Dreamy green eyes grin at me as she smiles, "I wish I could share this with you... one day... I promise... we'll go on a roadtrip... and eat lots and lots of shrimp."

She tells me of the elfish dance gone awry which led to a fractured vertebrae high in her back. Everything aches, but mostly her neck. Just a few months after her mother died, two rods were placed in Ruby's tiny back to help her sclerosis. Before alcohol, Ruby had grown addicted to morphine, turned into a tiny monster, and was sent to New York to live with her father and stepmother, both of whom she'd never met. From ten to twenty years of age, my best friend's story reads heavily, with abuse, months spent in hospitals, and bullies. I never met anyone my age whose tales outweighed mine, and I respect her for the long Holocaust she survived.

Living my whole life to relate to people, but learning from them as well, brings me the greatest companionship. In boyfriends I have not found the happy surprise of love and real education, but in Ruby I have. Despite all the fights we have about her drinking. Even after the times she's been drunk and hit me in front of friends because she thought I was competition for some ex-rockstar. While under the influence, Ruby has stolen money out of my wallet. She's been caught drunkenly pilfering a coatroom for cash. She has stomped on my iPod, said incredibly cruel things to provoke my tears, and gone after the guy I liked just to spite me. But this is all what she does while drunk. Sobriety makes her the crankiest, most illuminated creature I've ever known, but for many reasons she cannot stay sober. Like a battered wife, I trudge on hoping we'll get better.

An ER nurse informs us of the possibilities. Ruby may be bedridden for months. She may be stuck in a brace until next year, or the worst possibility, Ruby may need surgery. Rube and I talk about our options. They are "ours" instead of just "hers" because I am in it with her for the long haul. I can move back in and split her rent, caring for her when I am not at work. We will buy a futon and do our damnedest to find space apart so as not to kill each other. As we talk about this, I grow nervous. So nervous I want to cry. I cannot live without space, but she cannot live on her own under these circumstances. Realizing there are few boyfriends I would have done this for, I take my cell phone to the lobby where I cry for the first time to our West Coast friend. He is barely sympathetic and treats me as though this is my role. Maybe he is right, but I hang up hating him.

Back at bed 12, I sit at the head of her gurney, playing with her long, black hair.

"Why'd they take your underwear?"

"They made me take a pregnancy test. I told them I'm not pregnant! Why don't they ever believe you? What, do I look like a slut? Just 'cause I was dancing on bar..."

We are laughing far too much for a duo with a broken back, but laughing is what we do best. On each side of us are vomiting men, thankfully hidden behind curtains. As they spew in stereo, Ruby's eyes widen to silently tell me this is hell.

After two different homeless men occupy bed 14, I feel less guilty about my absence at my best friend's bed. One tells the doctor he smokes a pack of cigarettes a day and lives in the nearby shelter. The other is on methadone but used to be on heroin. In and out of the hospital on coffee, bathroom and cell phone breaks, I am just as scared but better than a person without someone to love this much. I miss a whole day of work to hold Ruby's cup of ice chips and her hand.

"I wish these chips were barbecue-flavored."

Rube had a CT scan before I arrived which revealed the fracture. We waited hours for the MRI. They would not allow her to eat, just in case. Just in case they had to perform surgery. It was 8 P.M. when we finally came back to the ER, after a traumatic MRI for claustrophobic Ruby, now stashed in bed 14. Should that make me nervous? Ruby gets frightened. She has cried a little off and on now. But not me. I won't cry yet, not even out of her sight. I tell her the MRI is gonna come back fine. In a few minutes they will suit her up in an ugly brace, we will hit a nearby diner for her bacon cheeseburger, pick up some prescriptive painkillers at Walgreens, and then we'll catch a cab home. Ruby and I are discussing what movie to rent that evening when the specialist returns with a foreign man in a nice suit. His accent is almost French. He will be operating on Ruby as soon as she signs the consent forms. I did not expect to be right or wrong in my predictions, but I knew what she wanted to hear so I said it.

As we listen to their plans, Ruby and I hold hands and tear up. The bad news: They will fuse her spine in about an hour. The good news: She will be fine in a few days. But there are consequences. Everyone knows the consequences of surgery to the spine. Doctors have to say them anyway. I get really scared, but it's nothing compared to Ruby. She was four pages into writing the story of her back surgery from childhood and cannot believe this is coming now. She knows all the terms for the injury after researching her seventeen-year-old operation. It is too much.

Upstairs we meet the team that will reassemble my mess of a friend. Like astronauts in an awful end-of-the-world-meteorite movie, they suit and scrub up. The surgeon will now open up and repair my most favorite creature. I put Ruby's cap around her mane as she tears up and finally asks, "What if I die?"

I hold Ruby's hand tightly and muster my lot. "It's gonna feel like fifteen minutes have passed. I will be seeing you as soon as you wake, and you'll be sore but you won't be dead."

She asks more what-ifs and just before they wheel her into the surgery room, I lean into her face and say two truths.

"Ruby, I know I will never die in a plane crash and I know you are not going to die tonight."

I kiss her forehead and they take her away as she sweetly says in her husky little voice, "I love you, Angie."

I walk down 14th Street at ten o'clock on Friday night, passing Beauty Bar and all the happy, beautiful people, carrying a clear plastic bag that reads, "Personal Belongings." In that bag are deadly shoes, a purse with a New York driver's license, torn red corduroy Dickies, and Ruby's cell phone. It feels like my feet are melting into the pavement or the pavement is melting into me. It feels like clocks have stopped. It feels like she is dead. She is not dead. She is lying open like a stubborn jewelry box, exposed but in good hands. I trust these people. I have to.

The A train gets me home where my suitemates are throwing an enormous party packed with self-conscious medical students. Unbeknownst to me, my bed and belongings have been stashed to make room for healthy young bodies. Everyone offers me a drink as I scramble to collect necessities. My day feels like something running all weekend on the Independent Film Channel. This is hell. I need a time out.

With a glass of champagne in hand, I duck into the storage room where my bed accompanies a stranger's pet Chihuahua. I call my mother and brother with drink in one hand, love-starved puppy in the other, and I cry a little. I laugh too. I really needed to find that spot.

Moments later I escape to Queens in a taxi shared with old friends on their way downtown. I laugh a lot with them. More than anyone in the world, I imagine. In Queens I pack Ruby's suitcase, throw my body around to happy music, shower, then pass out in her bed. At 3:30 A.M. the French doctor calls to tell me the good news.

"She did fine. We had to work around a lot of the bone. The rods had grown imbedded..."

She is fine. She did exceptionally well. That is all I need to know. She will be knocked out until noon. I call her mother and she shares my sleepy happiness. At 8 A.M. my phone rings again and Larry, part of Team Ruby, tells me she is doing really well. He tells Ruby I am on the phone and she shouts like a little girl, "Hi Angie!"

With a heavy suitcase, I meet Ruby in recovery. She is well. She is suffering though. I set up shop with laptop and bagel next to her as she pops in and out of sleep.

"That MRI was so scary. I kept opening my eyes and seeing weird people poking out of it. I was hallucinating from all the medication."

She is better but worse today. She is healing, though.

"My dad's not coming, right?"

"No, just your mom."

"Right. He hates hospitals and he can't leave the dog alone."

My sympathy pains increase with this news. Or I have been on the laptop too long. A Russian nurse hands Ruby a breathing contraption and she wears herself out puffing, then groggily asks the nurse, "More?"

The nurse walks away saying, "Yes, Ruby, more. More, Ruby!"

Rube mumbles at the nurse's back, "I wish you would forget my name."

I have wanted to be outside in the summer air, but someone I love needs somebody and for her I do not mind being needed. But don't pity me. I am the most selfish and unselfish girl. I do nothing that makes me unhappy except showing up at menial jobs for paychecks. Twelve hours is a long time to spend in a hospital, but not a long time with Ruby.

"Ang, remember that day… We were in my room… You were crying 'cause of Tommy… And then we ordered a pizza?"

"Yeah."

"That was fun."

And so is this. In its own screwed-up way.

Angela Lovell is an award-winning playwright, director, screenwriter, essayist, podcaster, writing instructor, film/music/theatre critic, performing monkey and soon-to-be novelist. After dropping out of New York University's Tisch School of the Arts, Angela wrote for Universal Studios and MTV. This year you can see her skewed "feminist" play *Self-Help* Off-Broadway, and her short film *Girl's Best Friend* at The Brooklyn Underground Film Festival. Angela lives in Brooklyn where she enjoys petting strangers' dogs and writing about herself in the third person.

Part IV

I didn't think there was a bottom deep enough to contain me.

I sat on the phone in tears...

"I need help—can you help me?"

The Path Was Rocky (But Worth It)
Steven Michael Sarber

Sobriety is different for everybody, and so it is hard to put into words what it feels like to have reached such an awesome goal after so many setbacks. But I will do my best.

My path to sobriety was rocky, and full of detours. I lost my way often and often stayed lost. I am sober now. Not "dry" or "on the wagon," but sober. That is one magical word. Sobriety. While in active addiction, it feels like the most unreachable goal one could ever dream of.

While I was drinking, I never—not once, not for a fleeting second—believed I could ever *be* sober. The most I ever hoped to accomplish was the illusion of sobriety. In truth, I would suffer panic attacks if the night was nearing a close and I hadn't found any money for alcohol. I sold everything I could to buy beer: guitars, my wife's CD collection, whatever wasn't nailed down.

Now, looking back, my degradation saddens me. But it shaped me into who I am. Today I like myself. Today my wife and son love me more than I probably deserve, considering the things I did when I drank. I was hateful, self-centered, rotten. I only thought about, cared about, drink.

At twenty-one, I received my first DWI. My blood-alcohol content was .284. I never fully understood what that meant until I was in rehab. A counselor explained to me that my blood was twenty-eight percent alcohol. Twenty-eight percent! And I was out there driving. It was appalling, but I also wore it as a badge. It was the highest blood alcohol level of anyone I knew.

It took four more DWI's, a near-divorce, and more than fourteen months' total prison time before my eyes finally opened. I missed my son's second and fourth birthdays. I missed Christmas and Thanksgiving dinners; I missed a whole lot of important things I took for granted anyway. I still wasn't learning. I cared, but not enough to change.

During what I thought might have been a real good attempt to become a sober man, I suffered pulmonary embolisms: three blood-clots in my right lung. I was twenty-eight at the time. The day I got out of the hospital, I bought a bottle of vodka. I didn't need the excuse; I would have drunk anyway. I wasn't ready yet.

I hid my drinking from my wife for about four months, then I drank openly in front of her. It was like a slap in the face to her, and that was when she began to fall out of love with me. I still hid my drinking from the rest of the family and I felt terrible when they would tell me how proud they were of me.

Finally, I went back to prison after violating my probation. When I shipped out to my state home, it was truly a godsend. I hadn't known my wife was falling out of love; she told me over the phone the day after Christmas. I cried. In front of eighty some-odd hard cases, I sat on the phone in tears. What did I expect? That she would let me walk all over her forever? That getting evicted from three apartments, having our power shut off on more than several occasions, having most of our friends not even want us around, that none of that should matter to her?

I had never cried in front of her and she realized a change was coming over me. I was finished. I couldn't live like this anymore.

She agreed to keep an open mind, and to see how things would be when I was released from prison.

I immersed myself in recovery. I spent all possible time in A.A. and N.A. groups. The prison I was serving time in happened to have the most groups of any prison in the state of Missouri. It was exactly where I needed to be at the time.

I gave my addictions over to God, and my cries for help were answered because I was ready to help myself.

Now, my ideal day is a sober one. I spend time with my son. I see my wife when she gets home from work. Then I go to work in the evening. It is not exactly a perfect arrangement, but it works for us. I write when I get home from work, and every night when I go to bed, I thank the Lord for another sober day. Then I ask for the next day. I do it this way because it works for me.

The date of my last drink was September 29, 2005. At the time of this writing, I have been sober for twenty-one months.

I do not think I am unique. I do not think I am special (even if my family would now argue that point). I am loved and blessed. I have a wonderful system of support. I am still recovering, and it is great. I love the time with my son, who is now almost six. He does remember I was away for a while, and he knows it was jail. Thankfully, he was too young to remember me at my worst. Now, because of the path I have chosen, where doors were once closed, new ones are opening. My family respects me again, and that is a feeling I wouldn't trade for the world.

I am thankful for every day for my life, and for my sobriety.

Born and raised in St. Louis, Missouri, the author has overcome many great obstacles to become a husband, a father and, perhaps most importantly, a sober man. He still resides in Missouri with his wife, Crystal, and son, Randy.

(continued from page 94)

Does Counseling or Therapy Help?

Absolutely! Counseling or therapy can help a person decide to get help, examine the drinking, stop drinking or make other life changes to support abstinence. There are many effective behavioral or psychosocial, medication and combined approaches for AUDs. These approaches may be used in any of the levels of care described earlier. Although the theory behind each treatment model is different and some of the clinical techniques vary, all aim to help the affected person manage the AUD and make changes in himself and/or his lifestyle.

Treatments that have been shown to be effective in studies sponsored by the National Institute on Alcohol Abuse or Alcoholism (NIAAA) include *cognitive-behavioral therapy, community reinforcement therapy, motivational enhancement therapy, motivational interviewing, relapse prevention, social skills training, social network therapy,* and *twelve-step therapy.*

(continued on page 127)

Amazing Grace
Dagan Elizabeth Manahl

I once was lost, but now I'm found. A little phrase that has inspired countless others and has a special meaning for me. I am not a particularly religious person, and I have always had a difficult time putting my faith in a "higher power." Who or what is this higher power? I always picture a vast presence in the sky, vaguely mechanical, not particularly human and not at all interested in the lives of us little folk down here. By definition it is an alien thing. I suppose for some people it is comforting to put their faith in some vast unknown, some idea that allows them to give over responsibility for their lives. But for me, by nature the one who always has to know "why," who needs the details of everything down to the last little particle, that is no comfort. I have found that people in general find this questioning quality a bit unsettling, or irritating, but I can't help it, it is who I am. But, Amazing Grace? I *know* that. That idea I can wrap my mind around. I once was lost, but now I'm found. No truer words have been spoken in the English language.

I was born to parents still living out their 60's dream, or nightmare, depending on what day it was. My mother was beautiful and crazy. Crazy as in one never knew if she was going to hug you or hit you, whether she was going to get out of bed or stay under the covers, crying for days. Crazy as in bona fide cannot function in society crazy. My father is a Vietnam veteran, and he does not speak of his time there, or much about his time married to my mother. I know some things are just too painful to talk about, but for a child born into this situation, it's like your childhood has been erased: no memories, no photographs, no rites of passage. You are born, and then *voila*, 20 years later, you are an adult, kind of like Athena sprung from the head of Zeus as a full-grown woman.

My parents were addicts. I am not talking about the nameless shuffling, sniffling, unkempt and skinny addicts you see in every inner city, but highly functioning, suburban-dwelling, secret-stash addicts. Some of my earliest memories are of the "dope man" coming round the house, bringing drugs for my parents. Then the door to their bedroom would close, and I would be alone. This was the pattern of my childhood. I won't dwell on that part too much. Through three states, countless years and as many houses, we traveled, my mother, my father and me. We finally landed in Colorado, where my mother—addicted, alone (my parents separated), hopeless, and hopelessly ill—took her own life. She left a note, but I could not hold onto that single piece of paper, with her long and elegant handwriting, slanting slightly to the right. It disappeared along with my childhood.

A child with no parents, no family to speak of, no life skills, very little education. Life is scary for a marginalized and powerless young girl. I coped as I knew how, by drinking. At first I was a social drinker, hanging out in parking lots with the other lost children (we *were* children), drinking 3.2 beer and singing along to Lynyrd Skynyrd or Led Zeppelin, depending on the night. Eventually, I left Colorado, bright with the promise of a long distance call from a father I barely knew, to come to Texas and get an education. Well, that didn't really work out for me, the father part. I did stay on in Texas, and continued to live my life in the familiar pattern of constantly moving from rundown apartment to rundown apartment, turning over newspaper machines for spare change when things got real bad, desperate for security and a better life, but never knowing how to go about getting some peace. Amazing Grace.

The years passed, and I can count them each by my choice of drink. The beer and wine cooler years of my adolescence, followed by the vodka and tequila years of my early twenties. Finally, the alcohol overdose years. I don't really like to think about those years. Amazing Grace, I lived on. Along the way I did manage to make it almost all the way through college, with the help of Uncle Sam and a bartending job (never far from the alcohol.) They say every alcoholic hits bottom, but let me tell you, I hit bottom, and bottom, and then bottomed some more. I didn't think there was a bottom deep enough to contain me. I tried to drive my brand new Camaro through a Dairy Queen. Literally. Amazing Grace, I walked away without a scratch, and drunker than any sane person has a right to be. I ended up in jail for public intoxication in my bra and a pair of bike shorts. Classy. I racked up $3,500 in unpaid traffic tickets, never bothering to show up for court. Did some jail time over that little situation. I made poor choices in friends, lovers, careers and lifestyle. Finally, I was at the point where I could only work every other night, because I would drink so much that I could not get out of bed the next day. I had to schedule my college courses around this same pattern: work and drink one night, recover the next day. I had chronic diarrhea and bruises all over my body, which I hid with body makeup and long jeans.

One day, a man walked into the bar I was working in. He was so quiet, thoughtful. When he left, he said "Here is my phone number, I hope you call me." I eventually did, and now we have been married almost ten years. Amazing Grace.

What can I say about those early years of our relationship? Do I count the times I went out and got drunk, and came home cursing at him, yelling that I hated him, that he was dirt, that I wished I had never married him? Do I count the times he patiently cleaned up after me, the vomit, the broken glass, the pain? Do I count the times he said "I love you" and "everything is going to be alright"? Eventually, I was forced to face my addictions by a judge. Ordered to attend five weekly A.A. meetings or violate and forfeit my probation—which I had already done once, by taking my sign-in sheet for A.A. and passing it around an icehouse off Interstate 10 in the heart of Houston, having all the drunks sign their names as I ordered rounds and cheered. When that didn't fly, my husband in desperation actually sat in on A.A. meetings, pretending to be me, getting my sheet signed to keep me out of jail. It was time to either get on with living, or put the final nail in my coffin. Amazing Grace.

Now, I don't much get along with the ideas of A.A. I don't have a lot of patience with folks sitting around rehashing and reminiscing about being a drunk, and how they've done everyone wrong. That is not my style. I know I did wrong. I don't need to tell a roomful of strangers to validate myself. We already talked about the higher power thing. However, there is one important thing that I did take away from my mandatory A.A. meetings, and it is the title of my essay, Amazing Grace. Amazing Grace that I conceived a child that year, a daughter. She was a happy and most fortunate event, because I finally understood what all the talking was about, what all the forgiveness was about, what all the pain was about. I also finally knew what loss was all about. Loss of selfishness, loss of the alcoholic I am and once was. I came home typically drunk exactly once after my daughter was born, to a crying baby, a frustrated husband whom I abused verbally and lashed out at, kicking and screaming that I hated him, and a long look in the mirror. A look in the mirror in the bathroom, which I woke up in, sick, smelly and ashamed. Amazing Grace. I once was blind, but now I see.

I would like to say I have not had a drink since that day, but I would be lying. Alcoholism is a lifelong disease for which there is no cure. Some days are better than others. Sometimes I can have a drink and I will be able to stop. Other times even thinking about a drink—a shot of smooth tequila with a lime or really good vodka—is enough to send my pulse racing and my palms sweating. Someone very important to me once told me that alcohol is like a unique poison to my system: while others can have a drink or two and continue to function, it poisons something vital inside of me, and it is a physical reaction. I have watched countless friends, acquaintances, family members and even strangers struggle with this disease. It is a disease that makes no distinctions based on age, gender, ethnicity and social status. The thing of it is, alcoholism comes in masquerading as a friend, a soothing companion, a choice. It becomes an enemy, the constant flattering companion that tells you it is okay to have fun, you deserve it, let your hair down, you are charming, witty, fabulous. Alcoholism is the same sly companion the next day, while you are nursing your splitting head, hating your illness, that tells you that you will never amount to anything, you are nothing, a failure. Alcoholism is a crawling need and a life destroyer, a killer, and a killer of potential.

I have two daughters now, a comfortable life in the suburbs. I drive the obligatory SUV and socialize with my neighbors at barbeques and block parties. I wear modest clothes and tone down my "shine." I say "shine" because shine is exactly what it is, the shine of overcoming, of conquering, of health. I drive into the city five days a week to my job at a conservative firm, a firm that has no inkling of the person I once was, the alcoholic. I look at my children, at my life, and I see what love can do, can be, manifested in another. The need to drink becomes a little less. Forgiveness a little nearer. Acceptance is a wonderful thing. Acceptance that I am powerless over this disease. Amazing Grace. How sweet the sound.

Dagan Elizabeth Manahl is a happily married mother of two and a recovering alcoholic who hides in plain sight. She dedicates this story to her husband for his unfailing support and patience, for not giving up or giving in, and to her beautiful daughters for teaching her how to be humble.

Losing Control
Jessica Saldivar

I have to be up in three hours to meet with my students, but I'm awake, tossing and turning. Where could he be? Should I even care about someone who puts me through this tiring anguish? Finally on the verge of sleep, the cellphone rings. It's him. He was driving—and drinking. My heart races and my stomach turns. "Heeey babbbee, where are you?" he slurs into the phone. Where would I be at three in the morning, besides being in bed and worrying about him? "I want to see you, but I'm lost!" he screams into my ear. Not another night of this, I think. It's late, I'm tired. But this night is different.

It was the day he lost his house in foreclosure. Thin, pale, only 28 years old and newly divorced, he looked like he hadn't slept in weeks. He hadn't. His life was spinning out of control. Creditors were hounding him; his memory was haunting him; his pain and depression were consuming him. Only alcohol and I consoled him.

She left him, his high school sweetheart of eleven years and wife of one. A new house, which she demanded, a live-in mother-in-law and a life of boredom had pushed her into the arms of another man. It crushed him. He was no longer who he once had been. now a lifeless shell, living for his next drink. And I was along for the ride.

Why did I stay? Why did I care for someone with so many problems? I was young, about to finish college. A chance meeting brought us together. So many possibilities, and I chose him. He had lost everything, including hope. I thought I could help. Imagine that.

"I don't know where I am!" His sobs broke through the phone. My heart is pounding. "They're going to get me!" he cries. He's referring to the police: he has no license, lost after his second DWI conviction. For a long time, I blamed the ex-wife. Who would do this to someone? Now I just blame the alcohol. He sobs some more. "Where are you?" I ask. Plead. Beg. Demand. He doesn't know. He can't tell me because he drank his sense away. I'm scared. What the hell am I going to do? I don't want him to be arrested. I think about calling the police myself. Would that be wrong? I start crying. That's all I can do.

He starts screaming again. I've never heard a man cry like this. I hear a noise over the phone. Has he hit something? I jump out of bed, frantic. What do I do? What do I do? I don't know where he is. "What do you see?" I ask. "Think!" I scream. "I wanna go home, babeee!" he cries, like a child lost in a store. He pauses—I can hear him sobbing, hitting his head, punching the steering wheel. Those bastards, his friends, how could they let him drive like this? I hate them. I hate them! Tears stream down my tired face. He slurs a description of a building he has just passed by. I hope he's where I think he is. I run out the door and into the car, half dressed and scared out of my mind.

I'm driving slowly. Crying. Looking and praying for some sign of him. I park the car near the Baskin-Robbins, right on the highway. I look crazy. It's 3:26 A.M. and I'm in my pajamas, searching for my drunken boyfriend. It's dark and cold and I'm so scared. I see a silhouette in the distance in an empty field. The figure is stumbling. Could that be him? I can't tell, he's so far away. What other woman would be out in a deserted field in the middle of the night in a dangerous city? I'm crazy! The figure falls; I hear a faint moan. It's him. I run as fast as I can in flip flops, the long weeds scratch my legs. My heart pounds wildly. I reach him. I cry even more. He's covered with mud. His eyes are bloodshot and wet, he looks puffy and broken. I love him. I love him so much. Why? Why? Why?

Stumbling uncontrollably, he has no idea what's going on. "Where's your car?" I ask. He doesn't know. He cries and I hold him up. Like always. He feels safe; I feel stupid and drained. The police come cruising by. I pray and hold my breath. I got to him before the cops did, thank God. This is the worst I've ever seen him. I feel so bad, ashamed, even embarrassed. What was I doing? How can I help him? I just keep picking up the pieces.

After a while of driving around aimlessly I finally find his car. A tire is flat; the door is wide open; the keys are in the ignition. But it's still there. Incredible! He passes out.

It was a close call. They all are, but this was the worst. How many more of these uncertain nights am I going to have to share with him? I want to run away, forget his problems. Forget him. But I can't. I don't. I want to help. I can help. Can't I? It would be easy to walk away. But I stay.

Jessica Saldivar is a 24-year-old law student and madly in love with Roman, who is struggling to put his life back together. Through patience, love, determination and perseverance, they beat the disease together.

To Drink or Not To Drink
Lisa Schoonover

If you have ever wondered if you've hit bottom, all I can say is, you'll know. Bottom is a one-two punch to the gut after giving karma the middle finger, mooning the Universe on a double-dare, diving into an ocean of fire, and knowing that no amount of bartering with the gods can take back the choices you've made. In other words, you're through.

My own private Idaho smacked me right between the eyes at approximately 12:54 A.M. in October of 2006, between a saltwater taffy shop and a cage-dancing club. I was arrested for DUI and although I wasn't driving, these days you don't have to be in order to earn yourself a free pass to the drunk tank. But I'm getting ahead of myself.

I began my night with wine-in-a-box and pizza bites. I was having a pity party over a recent breakup and listening to Nine Inch Nails. Suddenly, sparks of insanity fired in my limbic system and I devised a plan to drive to Cannery Row in disguise and hunt down the ex at his hangout. I dashed to my closet. Already in yoga sweats and an old T-shirt from a Police concert, I threw on a castaway Elvira wig and prepared for Operation Ex-out.

I guess I hadn't really planned on finding my ex, or what I'd do if I did, but alcohol has a funny way of tossing things like the decision-making process right out the window. Like that female astronaut who recently chased her lover down the freeway, I'd definitely hit an all-time low. Except I wasn't wearing a diaper.

I arrived on the Row and parked my new Nissan, pulling back and forth in the space until it was perfectly parked. I walked to a pub, ignored the snickers, and threw back a couple of Long Islands. Roughly an hour later, I left. Walking through the doorway, Fate shoved me right into the ex. He took a step back and stared at me in shock, his mouth hanging open wide enough to catch flies. I played it off like it was perfectly normal for me to cruise the Row in a Mistress-of-the-Dark wig.

But before my saturated forebrain could calculate my next move, we were tag-teamed by two officers. Funny thing about luck, after they checked our ID's, I was the only one given the sobriety tests. The police took their time, having fun at my expense, and finally cuffing me. They let the ex go. For the second time that week, he walked away without looking back, leaving me alone with my humiliation.

Why did they arrest me when I wasn't driving? A limo driver had called in a citizen's arrest after he watched me park, stating that I was rocking the car back and forth in the space.

He also claimed that he'd seen me trying to unlock my car door and that was what earned me a DUI with intent to drive. It didn't help that I blew a 2.1, well over the legal limit. I later found out he had lost a sister to a drunk driver.

I was taken to the Monterey police station. The police ran a background check and dug up an old misdemeanor, and high-fived each other. I would be held overnight without bail and charged as a second offender. I waited for over an hour and a half while I was booked, being treated like I was a degenerate criminal. My questions were ignored or met with hostility and threats. I was petrified and exhausted, and deeply angered. I was led to a holding cell with a broken toilet and no water. A bed made of concrete was covered with a thin, dirty foam pad. The air was stale and cold. Freezing and defeated I wrapped up, deep in my despair. I was never allowed a phone call. An old man in the cell next to me cried out in pain. Somebody banged on the bars and yelled at him to shut up. Every couple of hours I was "breathalized" until my blood alcohol level fell below .08. It took until 4:30 the next afternoon.

I'm now in an 18-month multiple-offender program. Two hours a week, twelve of us meet for "group." We sit around a long table with a counselor and talk about alcohol. No one wants to be there but there's an unspoken camaraderie knowing we're all in the same boat. Six mandatory "education" classes are required where we watch videos about dried-up livers, brain damage, and out-of-control drinkers taking risks. There's also a 15-minute "face to face" with the group counselor. They check to see if you're learning anything from the program, and if you are paid up, then they tell you to try going to an A.A. meeting. On top of exorbitant court fines, we have to pay for the classes, processing fees, and a fun little program called "home confinement." The DUI world has its very own language of shame.

My confinement program will last for 39 days. I received one day of credit for spending the night in jail. An ankle bracelet resembling a racer's stopwatch is strapped around my ankle, tracking my movements to and from the house. I work from home so group is the only time I'm allowed out. My probation officer comes by for surprise visits to make sure I'm here. But the really fun part is the monitoring system. A camera resembling a cable box is hooked up to a router and your telephone. When the phone rings, you turn the camera on so they can see you, then you get to blow into a breathalyzer. They can call you any time. And the equipment never works. Last week my camera caught on fire. In a year I'll have to pay to have an interlock device installed in my car, plus high insurance.

You may or may not have a drinking problem. This experience finally convinced me that I did and has at last gotten me onto the right path. Don't throw caution to the wind. Embrace it and learn from my life.

Lisa Schoonover is a successful author of poetry, short stories, children's books, essays and travelogues. Lisa is currently working on her autobiography and plans to take a spiritual journey around the world for her 40th birthday in June 2008.

(continued from page 112)

How Can Medications Help the Alcoholic?

Two different types of medications are commonly used to treat alcoholism. Tranquilizers (such as Valium, Librium, Serax, and Ativan), are used only during the first few days of treatment to help patients safely withdraw from the physical addiction to alcohol. The second type of medication (called *anticraving medications*), is used to help alcoholics remain sober and reduce their craving for alcohol. These include naltrexone and acamprosate. These medicines reduce the alcoholic's craving and contribute to improved sobriety rates and a decrease in relapse rates.

Another drug, disulfiram, serves as "aversive therapy" for alcoholics. If the alcoholic drinks with disulfiram in her system (it stays in the system for up to 14 days after the last dose), she becomes sick. This aversive reaction is a motivator for some alcoholics not to drink. The idea is to "buy the alcoholic time" so that she does not drink when craving alcohol. If she waits to drink alcohol until disulfiram is out of her system, there is a good chance that her strong craving to drink will have subsided. It does not increase sobriety rates or decrease relapse rates or cravings.

Naltrexone and acamprosate are the best choices for preventing relapse if used with together with professional counseling and participation in self-help programs such as A.A. Other medications such as topiramate and ondansetron have been shown to decrease drinking, but they are not approved by the U.S. Food and Drug Administration for the treatment of alcoholism.

Alcoholics may need medications for other medical or psychiatric disorders. Since some medicines used to treat these disorders can interact with alcohol, the alcoholic should always inform his physician about his alcohol problem. Also, some medicines, such as tranquilizers, have a high potential for abuse or addiction, so individuals with alcoholism should be vigilant about their use of these and work closely with their physician to limit the chances of becoming dependent on them.

(continued on page 133)

Buzz

Miriam Lee

I remember my first buzz vividly. I was seventeen and had scored a fifth of Jack Daniels through a friend of my boyfriend. To my amazement, I enjoyed the burn and was able to drink it right down without choking. Soon my legs felt light, I was happy and I had a lot to say.

By the time I finished high school, I had a whole new group of friends. Some were old enough to buy alcohol, and we had weekly parties. The night of my prom, I vomited in front of twenty people. That Fourth of July I barely noticed as a group of boys threw lit firecrackers at me.

I viewed my freshman year in college as a challenge: to drink as much as possible and still be able to party on. My dorm mates and I kept the empty bottles on display, trophies of our triumphs. See, no one really judged us in college. Everyone was doing it, or so it seemed. I managed to graduate with honors, but by my senior year I was drinking almost nightly. I convinced myself it wasn't interfering with my life, since I was making the Dean's List every semester. I was a born drinker and could out-party everyone I knew. I was proud.

After college, I found work easily at a major hospital. I got by: I never drank before work, well, at least I got a few hours of sleep before going in. But three years into my career I was accused of coming to work drunk. The stench of booze on me was strong and I could not easily get rid of it: I would shower at night and again in the morning and chewed gum most of the time. I told myself at the time that it was OK: I had just overdone it the night before and I wasn't "drunk" by morning. Looking back, I often didn't remember the drive to work. This behavior was not lost on my boss and I soon found myself on paid leave for "depression." But even this didn't curb my drinking for long. I told myself I just needed to start and stop my binges earlier.

I would get home from work at four in the afternoon and drink twelve to eighteen beers before going to bed at eleven. I needed it: I found myself in a very foul mood if I wasn't able to drink. I would even take beer with me when I drove back to my hometown. I felt invincible on the road. I knew I had a problem, but I didn't want to stop.

Soon I met David, the man I would marry. We met in a bar, of course. He had recently quit drinking and didn't give me flak about my habit. I didn't let on to him how much I was drinking, so when we made the decision to move in together, I was terrified. How could I hide it? See, I didn't mind him knowing I drank; I just didn't want him to know that I couldn't make it home without stopping to buy a case of beer for the evening.

I married this wonderful man who put up with all of my antics. We moved to my hometown and I started a new job. I was on night shift, so I found it easier to limit my drinking to the days I was off from work and I couldn't drink in the mornings. I wasn't an alcoholic, I thought, if I didn't have to start off my day with a drink! I was having a wonderful time at karaoke every weekend, making new friends at the bars, and being quite the social butterfly. Well, when I was drinking. When I was sober, I was depressed. I knew it, but I wouldn't admit it to myself. I truly hated myself.

Then one night my world came crashing down. I had begun taking an antidepressant drug in an effort to stop smoking: David and I were considering starting a family and I needed to stop some of my bad habits. I knew the drinking was going to be next, but I told myself I could stop easily if I had a good reason, like a baby. I was on "night shift time," and started drinking at about 4 P.M. David was in bed. I don't remember exactly how it happened, but I decided I could not live for one more moment; the thought terrified me. I was going to kill myself, and apparently I needed an audience. I woke David, told him what was going through my head and then ran off for a knife. I tried to shut myself up in the bathroom, but he was too fast for me. I don't know if it was the booze alone, but I suspect the antidepressant helped set me off. I was hysterical. I had a scalpel at my wrist and my husband was calling 911. He also called my mother, who showed up at my house at two in the morning. I was humiliated, but still convinced I wanted to die. This bought me a ticket to the emergency room, then the Behavioral Health Unit at the local hospital. The loony bin. Great.

We were able to convince the E.R. staff and the police to let my mother and husband drive me to the B.H.U. We stopped for biscuits on the way, and I felt OK. Maybe it was just going to be like a little vacation, I thought; it would certainly get me out of work. I knew then I didn't really want to die, but I still didn't want to stop drinking. I'd appease everyone for a while and then start sneaking around again.

It wasn't until Mom and David were stopped at the door of the B.H.U. that it hit me. They couldn't come in with me. I was told I'd be there for about a week. What?? No, no, that wasn't what I signed up for! But it was too late: I was committed and alone. This was my turning point. Alcohol had never really kept me away from my loved ones; I was terrified and wanted to go home. I knew right then that I never wanted to be there again.

I was given a detox regimen and kept in a room with a bed and a barred window. I shared a shower and bathroom with strangers. I was expected to go to meetings when all I wanted to do was sleep. I spoke to a therapist while there and told her I knew I didn't want to hurt myself or anyone else. And I didn't. I just wanted to leave. Not only did my mother and husband know what happened, but my father, stepmother, sister, and grandmother also knew. My grandmother didn't even know I drank! How could I face them again?

I spent a lot of my time there in prayer. Please God, I prayed, help take away this desire to drink, I want a second chance. Fortunately, my prayers were answered. It's been over a year and I haven't had the urge to drink. I can't believe how much clearer my head is now. I'm actually happy and I feel that my moods are mine. I'm more in control now. My family has forgiven me, but none of us has forgotten. I try now to set an example for others. It's amazing the difference a year without alcohol can make.

Miriam Lee is a freelance writer and the stay-at-home mom of a two-month-old.

(continued from page 128)

Recovery from Alcohol Use Disorders

Recovery is a process of accepting and managing the alcohol use disorder and making changes in oneself and one's lifestyle to reduce the risk of relapse. Recovery is a "self-management" process that also often involves getting support from other people with alcohol problems. Recovery is more than simply stopping alcohol use.

One of the major goals of treatment is educating and encouraging the person with the alcohol problem to become involved in a recovery process. While professional treatment is not a substitute for recovery, it often facilitates the person's involvement in a change process that extends far beyond the clinical encounter.

Recovery from alcohol use disorders involves changes in all aspect of one's life: physical, lifestyle, psychological, family and social. While some individuals are involved for a brief period, others are involved throughout their lives, especially those with more chronic and persistent forms of alcohol dependence. Recovery is viewed as an active process involving:

Learning information. Educating oneself about alcohol and alcohol problems, its effects on oneself and on the family, the role and limitations of professional treatment, and the processes of recovery and relapse.

Self-awareness. Understanding the impact of alcohol problems on oneself, one's family and others, and understanding how one is motivated to change, personal coping mechanisms, and personal barriers to change.

Coping skills. Developing or strengthening behavioral, cognitive, and interpersonal skills to manage the challenges of sobriety, and making changes to meet treatment goals.

Family or significant other involvement. Including others in treatment and the recovery process in order to reduce their burden, elicit their support, and provide them an opportunity to work through personal feelings and problems.

Self help programs. Actively participating in programs such as A.A.

Relapse. Anticipating and reducing the risk by being able to identify and manage relapse warning signs and personal high-risk factors.

(continued on page 140)

My Story
Yvette Fitzjarrald

I was born in Juneau, Alaska and was given up for adoption immediately after birth. Much later, my biological mother told me that my father was a heavy drinker who had threatened to hurt or kill me if she brought me home. The only family I've ever known adopted me when I was four months old.

When I was in the 4th grade, we left Alaska for Oregon, where Dad worked in the building business. I loved it in Oregon. We lived in the middle of nowhere. I had a dog, Pepper, who was my very best friend. My school was small—there were only eight other kids in my class! I was in heaven there, as much as a pre-teen/teen could be. I also loved high school. I started dating a boy who I really liked. But just when I thought things couldn't get better, my parents told me we were moving again! We moved back to Alaska during my junior year in high school.

Alaska seemed to have changed. Hardly any of my old school friends were sober. Most of the kids smoked dope and drank, even during the school day. Peer pressure took over, and I started doing those things too. I absolutely loved getting stoned. I always felt so giggly, goofy and relaxed when I smoked pot. Drinking was just as much fun. Looking back, I can't imagine living like that, but back then it was all I lived for. I loved being high, being drunk—being anything other than my boring, plain old self.

Soon after graduation, I met and married my first husband. We moved to Oregon together, where he began work as a mechanic. He was a drinker, much more hardcore than I was at the time, and he was stoned on drugs a lot as well. It was a source of tension in our new home, because I knew that once you got married and grew up you were supposed to stop doing those things.

I quit drinking shortly after I learned that I was pregnant with my first child. Even with as little publicity as there was on the topic back then, I knew that alcohol could damage my unborn child. Making the choice to quit was easy; doing it and living it was difficult. But I did eventually abstain, with only a few "relapses" after I realized I was pregnant. I gave birth to a baby girl.

I didn't pick up the bottle again until my daughter was about five years old. At that time, reality had sunken in. I was married to an abusive man who didn't love me. He didn't know the meaning of love any more than I did, since we were both alcoholics.

The feelings all came rushing back to me after that first sip, and I realized how much I had missed my old friend, the bottle. Drinking became a weekly occurrence. I'd go out on the weekend, without my husband, since one of us would have to stay home to watch the baby. By "going out" I mean drinking and running around with different men. I was a whore to anyone who would buy me a drink. My husband had his share of going out too. If I went out Friday night, he went out Saturday. He had his own life and own affairs. We continued that way for about six years. Not surprisingly, that lifestyle led to a divorce, and I moved back to Alaska.

I resumed the life I'd come to know and love. My life was spinning out of control and I couldn't see it. After two years of working, raising my daughter by myself (with help from my parents), drinking and doing various drugs, I'd hit an all time low. I began to contemplate sending my daughter to live with her dad. I'd been raising her alone; he'd had all this "freedom" to party. I wanted that freedom! Without my little girl in the picture, I would be free to live as I wanted to, party whenever I wanted and not have to worry about baby-sitters, or much of anything else.

But I ended up getting pregnant again. When I realized this, I tried hard to quit drinking. I would go to a bar, intending to drink just soda, but end up getting drunk. Finally I went to the local alcoholism counseling offices. I took a test there, to find out if I had a problem. The test results were a graph shaped like a "V." Scoring on the top left of the V meant that you are not a problem drinker. If you score down toward the bottom, you were. I ended up scoring down toward the bottom of the V.

I brought the test home and stuck it to my fridge with a magnet. I looked at it from time to time. But I continued to drink and smoke pot until I was about 4 months along in my pregnancy. Then one night my best friend, who I *think* is the father of my son, got very sick. I was so afraid that I called the alcoholism counselor. I was on the phone telling her how he needed to get help. She asked me, "Have *you* ever considered getting help?" I began to cry and I said, "I do need help—can you help me?" She immediately arranged for me to enter a treatment facility. That was December 28, 1991.

I've been sober ever since. I still miss drinking at times, or at least living like that. I miss being wild and free, with no accountability to anyone. I miss taking a break from reality and forgetting that I ever had problems. I know how it feels to want to just forget about life, if only for a day. For me, drugs and alcohol were the only way to kill the pain.

But I know that if I were to relapse, it would probably kill me. It would be a slow form of death. I'd lose everything that is important to me. Knowing that is enough to keep me sober. Sobriety is "life on life's terms." That's how I strive to live my life.

Soon after I got sober, I began to experience the emotional pain that I'd covered up while drinking. Things that I'd buried and forgotten resurfaced, ugly things that hurt me badly. Often, when it hurt badly, I would cry and call my counselor. She would talk me through it. I survived. I felt tattered and torn when these things would come up, but I got through them.

My precious son, who is now almost fourteen years old, suffers because of my drinking. Three years ago he was diagnosed with fetal alcohol syndrome. He has also been diagnosed with attention deficit disorder, which is secondary to his alcohol exposure. He is very difficult to deal with at times. He has also been diagnosed with mild cerebral palsy, an anxiety-depressive disorder, and obsessive-compulsive disorder. F.A.S. kids often have multiple diagnoses, and Tyler is no exception. Parenting him can be an arduous task.

I've somehow managed to get through that, and continue to fight for him today. I'd like to think that by being open and willing to talk about our story and my life I will be able to help others who are facing similar situations. By getting sober and teaching my own kids about the dangers of drinking while pregnant, I hope to be able to break the cycle of addiction that started with my father.

Having a strong support system of friends and family and a spiritual life is important to guarding against relapse. Sobriety consists of learning new coping mechanisms so that when those uncomfortable and painful feelings come upon us, we can deal with them instead of drowning them.

It is painful to admit that I caused my son's birth defect. It makes a lot of people uncomfortable, especially those who won't take the time to get to know me and those who are outraged that I harmed my own child. But I won't stop talking about it because the people I've helped far outnumber those who can't accept me for who and what I am.

Born in Alaska, Yvette Fitzjarrald now lives in Washington State with her paramedic husband and three children where she runs a dog rescue group covering the eastern part of the state.

(continued from 134)

Factors Affecting Recovery

The process of recovering from alcoholism and related disorders is affected by many factors, including: (1) the severity of the alcohol problem; (2) the effects of the problem on health, daily functioning and relationships; (3) the level of acceptance of the problem and need for help; (4) the individual's personality and cognitive abilities; (5) family and social supports; (6) the existence of therapeutic alliances with professional caregivers; (7) the appropriateness of the treatment plan; and (8) the demographic characteristics of the individual (age, gender, employment status, ethnicity). For example, alcohol dependent individuals with low levels of motivation to change are more difficult to engage in treatment or recovery than those who are motivated to change and want to get involved in recovery. However, this does not mean they cannot be engaged in recovery, as many unmotivated alcoholics eventually "hook" into recovery and make significant changes in their lives.

(continued on page 150)

My Demon
Mary C. White

It is so easy to fall into the trap of being a party girl. I thought I was loved and needed by the people in the bars. And I never believed I was an alcoholic. I believed that word was made up by people who just thought drinking was morally wrong or were afraid of what drinking might do to them. But I was wrong about all of it.

Alcohol held me in its grip and would not let me go. At first, drinking for me was just a part of socializing, but then it took over my life, controlling my mind, creating a person that was not me. I lived for Friday nights, for parties and time with the gang. My Fridays lasted until Saturday. Eventually, they lasted until Monday morning. I missed work, which prompted me to try cutting back, but I suffered from withdrawal and the sweats and pain were too much to bear. I vowed no more alcohol, yet always inside me I could not wait for Friday to come.

Alcohol turned me into an easy woman. After a couple of drinks, all I wanted to do was drink more and have sex. I didn't care with whom. I became the bar tramp. I was an easy mark and woke up many mornings wondering where I was. Even this didn't stop me from drinking. The worst part of my addiction was what it did to my daughters. My sweet girls became afraid and ashamed of me.

Thank God I never got violent with them. Causing them grief and the shame of their mom being a "party girl" was enough.

More than once alcohol tried to seduce me into ending my life. I fought, was involved in disputes with neighbors, and almost got arrested. I spent time in the psychiatric wing of the local hospital. I attended groups, had private sessions and vowed time and again to stop. Yet no one could reach me.

My anguish ended with a guardian angel, an angel I felt but never saw. One night during a weekend binge, the people I was drinking with started to fight. Of course, under the influence, I decided to join them. That's all I remember. I woke up the next morning in my own bed, lying in my own vomit. My head was reeling and my leg felt like it was on fire. I sat up and winced. I could not move my leg. Removing the blankets, I discovered that my right ankle and foot were twice their normal size. I had to swallow my pride and call my oldest daughter. When she came, she said nothing to me, dialed 911 and left. I went to the hospital. My ankle was broken and had to be set. If it did not set right I would possibly need two pins and a rod put in its place. I was discharged, sent home on crutches with an appointment set for three days later. At the follow-up, the doctor informed me that no pins or rods would be needed. I was so relieved I thanked God and cried my eyes out.

I found out later what had happened to me. I'd been attacked by the children of so-called friends when I refused to give them more booze. My daughter knew where I had gone and decided to check up on me. She took me home and left me in my bed. Amazingly, she never told me this story herself. When I asked her about it she replied, "I didn't think it would do any good to tell you, Mom, because all you want to do is party and drink." That was my wake up call.

From then on, every day I started out a little shaky, wanting a drink, but refused to take one. Instead I prayed. My faith gave me the courage to go to A.A., where my healing started, where I found true friends. I left meeting after meeting crying for redemption from this evil.

My tears, prayers and meetings have worked. I have been clean and sober for three years. My weekends are now spent writing. I have had short stories published and I have a publisher interested in my novel. I am still an alcoholic, but one proud to have beaten the demon that once held me fast.

The oldest in a family of nine children, Mary C. White is the published author of several horror stories and poetry.

Part V

*I will never forget the sight of him stepping
through those metal doors...*

The promise to be everything I could be was still inside me.

One step at a time...
he is *learning to live*.

The Wake Up Call
Sheri Ables

I am almost the ex-wife of an alcoholic. Almost. This is the second time I have filed for divorce from my husband. I cannot tell you the number of times my husband and I have separated. It has been a rocky road, but I had to wake up. I came to the point where I knew there was nothing else I could do; I had to move on with my life. Is this easy? Not at all. Am I happy? I am saddened that it has come to this, but I am happy to be out of the situation. I have learned that I am powerless to help my husband as long as he does not accept that he is an alcoholic. Alcohol has the power: the power to hurt and to abuse; the power to turn a great life into a living hell.

My wedding day should have been a warning to me of the problems to come but I had on my "new-love blinders." We were married by a Justice of the Peace in a neighboring state and on our way home before I had time to blink. Only we didn't go straight home. We stopped to pick up his daughter and a six-pack. Once home, I cooked supper; he drank beer. As the night came the arguments ensued. His daughter cried to be allowed to sleep with him (crying always worked for her). They slept on the couch together and I spent my wedding night alone in my bedroom. *Wake up, woman!*

As time went by I became ever more blind to the signs that were virtually slapping me in the face. Is it OK to let alcohol come before being there for your wife when her mother passes away? Is it OK that your son has major surgery and almost dies, but your husband is too drunk to drive to the hospital, and asks instead, to "let me know how it goes." Is it OK to swear you have had only one beer, but hide the fact that it was one 32-ounce?

Alcohol is the great excuse-maker; it dissolves the strongest of wills. The excuse-maker creates ways to make drinking OK. I learned to craft my excuses for the problems; I adopted many of my husband's excuses as my own: he is a hard worker; he is tired at the end of a long, hot day; he is consumed with stress; my disapproval of his drinking adds to his stress; my children add to his stress. And, of course, he does not have a problem with beer, he can quit anytime that he wants. And he would quit when he was ready, not because someone makes him quit. A few beers after work do not hurt; in fact, some doctors recommend a beer a day. *Hello woman...wake up...a beer a day does not equal a six-pack a day.* There is no physical abuse and that becomes another excuse: *at least he doesn't hit me. At least he drinks at home instead of staying in bars. If he really had a problem, he'd drink at work.* Are you tired of the excuses—his and yours? Is this the way you want to live for the rest of your life?

Maybe you know what I am talking about. Maybe there is someone in your life who wields alcohol's power. Let me tell you, that person is powerless—against alcohol. Alcohol takes over the life of its host. I pray that my husband wakes up before it is too late. It is already too late for our marriage, as it was for the two others he lost before ours. He has nothing to show for years of work except a stock of beer in the refrigerator. I do not want my children (or his) to grow up thinking alcohol abuse is OK, or that living in an alcoholic home is OK. It is not OK. It has taken a lot of time and heartache for me to understand this fact, but I finally do, and I am at peace knowing that I am working toward a better life.

If you are living in an alcoholic home, there *is* a better life. Take that step. Make the move. You will be so glad you did. And it may be the very thing the alcoholic in your life needs. Stop enabling and start taking the power into your own hands.

Sheri Ables is a freelance writer, editor and literary agent. She has been in the publishing industry for over fifteen years. In addition to her literary career, Sheri works with Ameriplan to help families obtain affordable health benefits. She is the mother of four and resides in Mississippi with her children, her cat and her rabbit.

(continued from page 140)

How Do Alcohol Problems Affect the Family?

A number of years ago, a colleague and I interviewed adult and younger members of the families of individuals suffering from AUDs about the impact of alcohol and other substance problems on individual family members and the families as a whole. The following quotes capture the pain of living with the disease.

The Experiences of Young and Teenage Children

"I worried about mom all the time. She couldn't cope with dad's drinking. He'd yell, cuss and hit her, too."

"It was embarrassing. I wouldn't bring friends home because I never knew if my mom would get drunk."

"I had to take care of my little brother and sister. If I didn't, who would? Mom just couldn't do it."

The Experiences of Adult Children

"It was sad. Mom and Dad got divorced because of Dad's alcoholism. I felt stuck in between because they were bitter with each other."

"For years, I desperately tried to get my dad's approval. But he never noticed or seemed to care about what I was doing. I don't think he knew what I studied in college."

"The guilt and shame were tremendous. I felt like something was wrong with my whole family. I felt inferior to others, like I wasn't as good as them. I still hardly visit home, the memories are just too painful."

The Experiences of Spouses

"I felt like I had to be both mother and father to our kids. I told myself I wouldn't let my kids suffer because their father was more interested in drinking than being with the family. No matter how much I gave the kids, they still were deprived because of my husband's alcoholism."

"Being married to an alcoholic is like not being married 'cause you can't depend on them. They make you feel like it's your fault they drink. Nothing I did would ever pleased my husband, but like a fool I kept trying."

"I got obsessed with my wife and constantly watched over her. I thought maybe I could prevent her from drinking. What a fool I was. My moods were dictated by her. In fact, my life centered on my concern about her and her drinking."

As these quotes show, the family unit as well as its individual members, no matter their age, may experience adverse effects from exposure to a person with an alcohol problem, particularly those with a low motivation to change or who display, poor judgment; violent, suicidal, homicidal, bizarre, or unpredictable behavior, or those whose functioning is severely impaired. Any area of functioning of the family member—physical, emotional, social, interpersonal, occupational, spiritual or financial—can be affected. The burden on the family can be great, and some members may experience serious depression or anxiety.

Treatment can help the alcoholic acknowledge and address the impact of the disease on the family. It can also help the family deal with an individual member's reactions to the alcoholic.

Support groups like Al-Anon can help the members in their own struggle to recover from the effects of living with an alcoholic.

(continued on page 164)

No Longer in Charge
Christine Valentine

Only thirty when my first husband died, I grieved deeply and awoke each morning after his death with an overpowering sense of loss and dread of what the day would bring. I didn't know how I could possibly cope with all the tasks and responsibilities that I now had. But I maintained my faith in God and decided to put my life in His hands. The effect was immediate; I found the energy, day by day, to do more tasks and slowly pulled my life together. Eventually I remarried, and it felt like I was in charge of my life again.

A few years later I began volunteer work at an alcohol detoxification unit on a nearby indian reservation. I drank every day, one before lunch, several before dinner and sometimes heavily at parties. I did not consider this to be a drinking problem, since everyone around me was doing the same, and some were regularly intoxicated. But the need at the unit was great, and I was eager to help. I chatted with the patients, encouraged them and drove them to nearby treatment centers. At one of these centers I met an old friend. When I last saw him, he'd lost his job, missing too many workdays due to binge drinking. Now he was sober and the assistant director of the treatment center. I asked him, "Do you think I ought to stop drinking, since I'm a volunteer?" He said, "It's up to you, but you'll have a lot more credibility with the patients if you abstain." That made sense to me, so I decided to quit drinking.

I tried. But under pressure from friends I found myself succumbing to drinking again. Sometimes I had a really strong craving for it. It perplexed me that I could not completely stop.

One day a patient asked me, "Do you ever drink alone?" I found myself lying when I answered no. But the truth was, I did drink alone. I took a couple of beers with me when I went fishing, and had a cocktail or two and a glass of wine with dinner when traveling alone. So what, I thought. So did others! I was constantly comparing myself to other people who were heavier drinkers than I was. It took a long time for me to realize that what counted was my personal relationship to the bottle, rather than other people's drinking habits.

I was ashamed about my lying. So one day, I sat down and filled out one of the tests used at the treatment center to gauge patients' drinking problems. A score higher than a three and there was a good chance there was a problem. I scored four! Of course, I immediately rationalized the whole test and pushed the results away, but as time went by it kept creeping back to nag at my conscience.

Eventually, I decided to take a pledge with the local minister to abstain for six months. In those days, it was a popular way to stop drinking. I was confident I would be able to keep a promise to God, but I did not realize how difficult it would be. I spent six months with white knuckles. I craved a drink. I was bad-tempered; I even had violent thoughts. But those six months were a blessing because I was able to recognize my addiction. I was suffering from what I had learned was "dry drunk": negative thought patterns that eventually lead to a "wet drunk": drinking again.

When those six months were up, I took another pledge, but this time I was humble. I was not trying to prove a point. I was asking God's help with a serious problem for the second time in my life. Just as before, I knew that my higher power would help me. My Indian friends taught me that a prayer is a commitment. So I joined a twelve-step group to get help. As I learned about the twelve steps, I realized that I had already completed Step Two: "Come to believe that a power greater than ourselves can restore us to sanity." But I still needed to start at Step One; to look at my denial process and admit my powerlessness with alcohol.

Twenty-five years later I am still sober. I have a husband of thirty years and four grown stepchildren, whom I love. I gained sobriety and happiness through my commitment to a twelve-step program, by turning things over to my loving and supportive higher power and placing him in charge of my life instead of trying to do it by myself. Although I know that I am getting stronger all the time, it is comforting to know that He is in charge of my life. I believe as I have heard so many times before, "With God, all things are possible."

After coming to this country from England in 1964, Christine Valentine married and settled in Montana, where she worked as a chemical dependency counselor for the Northern Cheyenne Tribe until she retired. Her writing has appeared in *Hard Ground: Writing the Rockies III & IV*, *Foreign Ground: Traveler's Tales*; *Voicings From the High Country*; *Wyoming Voices*; *Blessed Pests of the Beloved West*; *Crazy Woman Creek: Women Rewrite the American West*; and *Owen Wister Review 2006*.

A Mother's Journal
Susan Norton

September 8, 1983

What's happening to our family? Once, joyful giggles tripped over themselves, and togetherness was something to look forward to as we rushed through our lives. Now, on those rare occasions when we eat together, my stomach churns at the air of rebellion, the cold words, the bloodshot glares, the nasty remarks shot back and forth across the table in staccato time. My protestations are shackled by dread, aimed at a son I no longer know. I wonder, do other parents go through such things? Is this just a stage of growing up? Don't all kids rebel, experiment and then go on with life?

October 3, 1983

I pace the floor, a Bible shaking between my hands, a clutching Christian robed in apprehension, unable to read, the pages blurred by fear, unable to pray, able only to whisper the words, "Help us." Someone once said God has a special regard for the prayers of mothers. Why can't He hear mine? Helpless and hopeless, I wish that someone, somewhere, would heed my silent screams.

October 15, 1983

I slink into my car, cocooned within, feeling safe and sane for a few guarded moments. The sounds of Bach relax my muscles:

tight, twisted, unyielding. Suddenly, the tiniest feeling of joy creeps into my brittle heart. It startles me. Even fleeting happiness scares me so. It makes the despair of my reality seem that much harder to go back to. Instead, I choose to walk around on eggshells, waiting for the next emergency of motherhood, the next challenge to my coping skills. I consciously push that flutter of pleasure aside and resolve instead to opt for a shroud of numbness.

November 11, 1983

I hear a siren in the night. My heart stops. The sound of a helicopter nearby makes my breathing freeze. The telephone rings, my stomach clinches. I stand another solemn vigil through a long and solitary night, once more waiting for the child I used to know, afraid to ask for miracles, praying only for his safe return.

November 23, 1983

Who is this boy? I do not recognize the anger that spits from his mouth, the lifeless, empty stares glued on the face of this stranger. Those beguiling blue eyes that once laughed and charmed me so have gone dead. The mouth that once smiled has gone slack. Yet I know, as only a mother knows, that someplace inside this shell before me, my son still lives.

December 10, 1983

Should I search his room? Does he deserve the privacy to destroy himself? I'm afraid what I will find: liquor bottles, rolling papers, razor blades, mirrors, strange looking glass pipes. What do I do then? I think I'll simply close his door, turn away and pray a little harder. Perhaps, perhaps it will all go away.

December 21, 1983

'Tis the holiday season. I stand at cocktail parties, sipping soda water with lemon, my gaze lost in the glass, wondering about this hold of absolute evil upon my son. I smile sweetly at other mothers, as if my only worries are my son's college choices. Yet, while others stew and fret about their child's SAT scores, I silently pray that mine will simply survive this very night.

January 7, 1984

I am at lunch with girlfriends, daring to enjoy myself. The police call. They are holding him. He's on beer and Quaaludes. "Come and get him," they say. I bolt to my car, tears dripping down my cheeks. I do not bother to stem their flow. I keep repeating, "I don't care." It's not the truth, but somehow I need this mantra to keep my shell of a life from shattering completely. I am clueless as to what to do. From the police station, I take him directly to another psychologist, who says he must be getting mixed up with a bad crowd. "I've learned my lesson this time," my son says. There's a tear in his voice. I have to believe him, for my own sanity.

January 14, 1984

Waiting for the other shoe to drop while wearing vigilance like a cloak. That's how I spend my days and nights. If I give up my son is doomed, lost to a world of darkness. All I know is that I must keep trying to find the single word or phrase that could possibly penetrate his excuses, open him up, free his mind, his heart, his conscience. I'm not above intimidating, buying him off, humbling myself before the angels. It is my job as a mother to fix his world and see him smile again.

February 2, 1984

Where is he? He left so many hours ago. Running interference for him, shielding him from consequences, school officials and policemen has become my full-time job. I pay him to read drug pamphlets. I beg. I bribe. I threaten. After each disaster, I know he must have learned his lesson this time. But I'm not learning mine. I drive by his school to see if his car is there. I creep over to it and check the trunk for signs of illegal drugs. His life is measured in six packs, dime bags and grams. So is mine. The merry-go-round continues. Neither of us can get off.

May 5, 1984

This date is branded in my memory: the day he is hospitalized. I trick him by saying that he is only going to meet with another professional and then go on to school. I will never forget the sight of him stepping through those metal doors. They slammed with such finality; it sliced my heart open. I knew at that moment that he would never forgive me. I might have lost my son, but just maybe he will live to find and save himself. I question the intake counselor whether he really belongs here. He pats my hand and says, "I asked your son what he would say if I put some bottles of booze, a gram of coke and a baggie of grass before him on this table." He said, "I'd think I'd have died and gone to Heaven." I sign commitment papers with a hand that quivers, feeling drenched in fear and failure.

Professionals calmly speak of his addictions. Don't they know that he's my son? He's barely seventeen. He wears Polo shirts and designer jeans, has short hair, goes to dance class. My mother's heart cries out, "Not my child!" But my adult's mind acknowledges: it is so. The diagnosis plunges forward like a tidal wave: "Middle stages of alcoholism and drug dependency," they tell me. "He's headed on a dead-end course for disaster, and it's killing him." And it's killing me. Dear Lord, it hurts so very much! How can one so young conquer such a foe, spend a life without the chemicals that have become his best friends? I am tethered to pain, unable to escape, incapable of throwing it off. But how much heavier *his* must be.

I lock his bedroom door when I get home, unable to face the emptiness in both home and heart.

June 7, 1984

My son sits across from me, his foot tapping in beat to the butterflies in my stomach, and takes my hands in his.

"Get me out of here, Mom. With your help and God's help, I promise I will never use again." His eyes mist. His hands tighten, ever so slightly. His mouth turns up in the most innocent of smiles. He knows that the mention of God is like a rush of fresh air through my resolve. The professionals have warned me that "if his mouth is moving, he is lying." I want nothing more than to take him home, pretend this is not happening, and love him back to normalcy. But my well has run dead dry. "You have to stay," is all I can get past my lips. He surges to his feet. His fists are tight knots, drumming against his thighs, his eyes cold as stones as he slashes past me. I know cold fear.

June 16, 1984

On my first night at the hospital's parents' group, my voice quivers. "Don't try to say it's not my fault. Every cell in my body tells me it is." The rest of the evening I sit, hands buried in my pockets, mouth frozen shut. What a long road lies ahead. Recovery for both of us seems like such an impossible word. Old as it is, it seems like the journey has just begun. So many feelings come up. Why was I so blind to all the signs, so gullible, trusting, defensive, such a failure as a mom? Could I not have looked past his fierce demeanor, the bloodshot eyes, and seen instead the pleadings from those same eyes, his voiceless cries for help?

July 30, 1984

He's coming home, back to his reality as an alcoholic/addict into a swanky suburb of Los Angeles where the roads are paved with denial. What will happen? I only know that I can do nothing but enforce the rules of a contract we have hammered out between us under the direction of the drug program personnel. It may not keep him "clean" but it will keep me sane.

August 5, 1984

Where once a bottle opener hung, sobriety chips now dangle from his key chain: thirty, sixty, ninety days. One step at a time, like an infant learning to walk, he is learning to live.

August 10, 1984

They call it the Family Disease. They tell me I must let him go, cut the cord of maternal enabling, release him to his own future, whatever that may be, step away and no longer rescue him from himself. Trust is like a double-edged sword. I laugh to myself at the word. Like I would ever be able to believe him again? But slowly, tiny step after tiny step, he proves to himself and to me that he can be trusted, and hope makes its home in my heart.

August 27, 1984

Stories tumble from him. He tells me when he was first in rehab, he tried to cut his hand with a sharp piece of metal. He thought that if he hurt himself bad enough, they would have to get him into the regular hospital from which he could easily escape. What got his attention was the reality that he could not feel the slash of sharp metal against his skin. His hand was numb, a reaction to the drugs. It scared him and he thought, "Just maybe, I had better stick around and give this recovery thing a try."

October 19, 1984

Our language changes slowly. Words like "sober" and "clean" become buzzwords and mini-prayers. Slogans clutter our refrigerator door: *Easy Does It. Turn It Over. Keep It Simple. Live One Day at a Time*, they tell us. What a simple slogan. It rolls off the tongue so easily, slips like ice cream down your throat, but is so hard to do. Like a muscle is built up by exercise, the more we live this day alone, the easier it becomes.

November 28, 1984

Other grieving parents call, voices low and scratched with tears, their stories much the same as mine. I share experiences with them. Desire to help has replaced my pride. They know they are no longer alone. They have found a fellow passenger down a road, a road that is booby trapped by their children's addictions.

December 15, 1984

Kids, trapped by their abuses, come knocking on our door. They are welcomed into our lives. We see past their vacant glares, the litanies of excuses, the rosters of people they blame, their foul, belligerent mouths, and we simply love them until they can love themselves.

March 6, 1985

The past no longer plagues my waking hours. Nightmares are replaced with dreams. Future fears are dimming. Still, I know there is hope, not promise, in this day only.

May 5, 1985

He's one year sober today! He has his future back and so do I. Trust has slowly been rebuilt, brick by brick, kept promise by kept promise. He puts one foot before the other, following a yellow brick road towards tomorrow. Some days he skips, other days his path becomes steep with challenges. But overall, his destiny is of his own design. His life is in his hands, no longer mine.

May 5, 2006

Twenty-two years of sobriety. He has graduated from college, gotten a master's degree, has a job he enjoys and a family he adores. Like all of us, he's gone through the ups and downs of life, traveled highways that twisted and turned, some to dead ends, others to beyond the sun. The journey continues.

Published in over 70 literary journals, magazines, anthologies, newspapers, greeting cards, two art exhibits, a cruise brochure, a tear-off calendar, NPR radio and even fortune cookies, Susan Norton has received ten awards for her writing. With her writing partner, she has published a seven-book series entitled *Pyramid Pal's Adventures in Eating*. Her latest adventure is her foray into the world of travel writing.

(continued from page 152)

Why Do Alcoholics Drink Again?

Many different situations or factors can contribute to drinking following a period of sobriety. Drinking may be in the form of a "lapse" (a single episode of use that is stopped) or a "relapse" in which alcohol is used on multiple occasions over time.

It is usually a combination of factors that contribute to alcohol relapse. For example, an alcoholic at a restaurant or a party may respond to pressure from others to drink alcohol even if the pressure is subtle. Or, drinking may be an attempt to reduce anxiety or boredom and to feel part of a group that is perceived to be having fun. An alcoholic may drink mainly when upset and angry at a spouse following an argument because he lacks the coping skills needed to manage interpersonal conflict. Therefore, it is not only the "high-risk" situation that is a cause of relapse, but the alcoholic's ability to use coping skills to manage the situation. The most common factors contributing to relapse are negative emotional states, social pressure to drink, interpersonal conflict, positive emotions, and urges, temptations or strong alcohol cravings.

(continued on page 170)

Reason to Believe
Ginger B. Collins

It was a great party. The vodka gimlets waited in a crystal bowl, cradled in ice like oysters on the half-shell. I could snatch one from its frozen bath whenever I wanted—and I wanted often. That combination of ice, octane, and Rose's lime slid down my throat, filling all the jagged crevices along the way, until I felt warm and smooth inside and out.

Then I woke up, jostled back to my reality as a fifty-year-old woman who had been sober for almost one year. True to my stubborn nature, I had gone cold turkey when the diagnosis of a thyroid condition collided with my life as a functioning alcoholic. I was determined to end my love affair with alcohol and never look back, and replace the hunger for a drink with a righteous desire to say, "I did it all by myself." I was pigheaded enough to pull it off—until my subconscious stepped in.

My therapist had told me about dream drinking. She described it as God's way of telling me that the craving wasn't gone, it was just hiding. I knew she was speaking the truth, but as I drove to my weekly appointment, the pros and cons of full disclosure played tug-of-war in my mind. I sat in the parking lot watching the digital clock run out the last minutes before my session. I knew that if I told her about the dream, she would bring up a subject I had avoided for months.

"You look chipper today," she said, leading me into her office to my regular spot in the overstuffed floral chair in the corner. It was from this flowered perch that we regularly peeled away the layers of armor that guarded my true feelings and chipped away the old beliefs that no longer served a good purpose. I had climbed to higher levels of consciousness from this chair, and I now felt myself poised to take another step.

"I look chipper because I feel chipper," I said. "Nothing like a good night's sleep." I chuckled at the irony. "And, this morning I made a big decision."

"Yes?" She settled into her chair with my file on her lap and a pen in hand.

"You know how I whine every time you mention A.A. meetings? Well, I've decided to go to one."

"Excellent."

"Don't get me wrong. I still don't want to go. But I had a drinking dream last night. It seemed so real, and the vodka—I could taste it. It was heavenly, but I know it's a sign."

"A message from God, sent through your subconscious."

Her words were followed by a smile. Not an "I told you this would happen" kind of smile, but a positive beam that showed her pride in my admission that I shouldn't fly solo. Patience was her strong suit. She had never told me to stop drinking. Even when the thyroid condition made it a wise choice, she waited it out. Instead, she dug into other problem areas and let me solve the alcohol dilemma on my own. Now, knowing that the time was right, she reached into my file and pulled out a paper.

"You'll need this," she said, and handed me a list of local A.A. meetings.

I decided on a Ladies Only meeting in a neighboring community, hoping for an extra measure of anonymity. The attendees were a cross section of American women: career types in well-tailored suits sitting next to college girls with backpacks. A little old lady with a lapful of yarn talked to the young mother beside her. The mother rocked her sleeping baby while the knitting needles clicked in rhythm. It was a group of women with nothing and everything in common. The topic for discussion was "The Big Lie," and there was no shortage of comments.

"I lied to myself all the time," said one woman. "Told myself I was still in control—that my drinking had no effect on my work or my kids." Her words connected. Heads bobbed in agreement and a few shouts of "Amen, sister!" percolated from the back row, creating the feel of an old-time revival.

Then the meeting leader spoke. "Rod Stewart had a song in the seventies. It was titled 'A Reason to Believe.' I think of it when I realize that life in a bottle doesn't work. We know it doesn't work, and we know there is a better way to live. But we still look to find a reason to believe in the next drink."

That bit of Rod Stewart transported me to the mid-seventies and the relationship that reshuffled my priorities and made it easy to turn drinking from a weekend vice into a daily habit. I remembered that man, and those years. I was chilled to think how easy it had been to stand at the fork in the road and make the wrong choice.

It was 1971 and I was a twenty-three-year-old mother of a young daughter. With the ink barely dry on my divorce papers, I returned to my home town looking for a new start. That's where I met Ray. He was tall and blond, with a prowling presence and denim blue eyes that could melt your heart and drop your pants with one look. I knew his history—ladies' man, party boy. I didn't care. To me he was the sweet relief for my bruised heart and deflated self-image.

We lived, loved, and never missed a party. When the dust cleared three years later, I eased my broken heart with the other remnants of our time together—a fabulous recipe for Bacardi Cocktail and the ability to pick Chivas Regal in a blind taste test. My relationship with Ray was over, but my relationship with drinking was not. Alcohol had woven itself into the fabric of my daily routine.

The Rod Stewart song always reminded me of Ray. It so aptly described our years together—the heaven of the first two years, followed by the lying and cheating of the third. He would look at me with those haunting blue eyes and tell me there was no one else. I wanted it to be true, so I told myself it was. It took years to realize the love affair with him was just like the love affair with alcohol. I knew drinking was bad for me. But I lied and told myself it was just an innocent buzz in the afternoon, a way to relax at the end of the day. I looked to find a reason to believe.

Sitting in that first A.A. meeting, it all came back to me. I remembered how I stumbled into alcohol addiction with my eyes wide open and spent years refusing to see its effect on my life, my family, and my soul. I was grateful for the dream that pushed me to this place, and thanked God for the reality check. I prayed for each woman who shared her story and her ordeal, and I asked God for strength to keep me alert and on course as I took sobriety one day at a time.

When the meeting was over, I headed for the car. Halfway through the parking lot I reached for the cell phone, eager to share the experience with my therapist. Just as I was telling her about the meeting, the song, and all the memories it rekindled, I turned the key in the ignition and the radio came on. Yes, it was Rod Stewart's familiar rasp:

"If I listen long enough to you, I'd find a way to believe that it's all true."

Ginger B. Collins is a published author of creative non-fiction that focuses on life, liberty, and the pursuit of happiness. Her "slice-of-wave" sailing tales have appeared in *Cruising World Magazine* and *LivingAboard Magazine*. Both *The Atlanta Journal Constitution* and *The Cincinnati Inquirer* have published her travel articles in their Sunday Travel Sections, including a two-part story in the *Inquirer* about a trip to China in the middle of the SARS epidemic. Ginger is Vice President of the Atlanta Writers Club and co-founder of the Brush Creek Writers' Cooperative. She lives in Atlanta with her husband, Melvin.

(continued from page 164)

Can an Alcoholic Reduce the Risk of Relapse?

Relapse prevention (RP) strategies focus on key issues associated with relapse and long-term recovery. RP strategies help the alcoholic prepare for the possibility of relapse and therefore reduce relapse risk by: (1) identifying and managing individual high-risk relapse factors; (2) identifying and managing early warning signs of relapse; (3) intervening early should a lapse or relapse actually occur; and (4) making broader changes in order to achieve a more balanced lifestyle so that alcohol is not desired.

Identifying and managing high risk situations. Anxiety, anger, boredom, emptiness, depression, guilt, shame and loneliness are the most common emotional factors contributing to alcoholic relapse. Interpersonal situations such as direct or indirect social pressures to drink alcohol or conflicts with another person are the second and third most common causes of relapse. The alcoholic can reduce relapse risk by first examining which emotions or interpersonal situations are perceived to be high risk for relapse. Then, specific strategies can be learned to deal with these high risk feelings and situations. For example, the anger problems of one individual may require learning to accept and express anger appropriately. Anger problems for another may require learning to control anger and rage, and not express it in interpersonal encounters. Boredom for one individual may be a function of lacking interesting hobbies or activities whereas with another, boredom may represent a serious problem in a job in which this person feels underused, underemployed, and not challenged.

Identifying and managing relapse warning signs. Both obvious and subtle warning signs often appear prior to an alcohol relapse. For example, lowered motivation may be indicated by an increase in negative attitudes toward recovery or A.A. Another common warning sign is putting oneself in high risk situations such as socializing with old drinking partners. A person may not be consciously aware of a relapse "setup," so alcoholics should learn common relapse warning signs and ways to manage them. Those who have had previous relapse experiences can learn to analyze these experiences in order to become aware of the warning signs that were ignored in the past. Family members can play a helpful role by pointing out warning signs they've observed before past relapses and by agreeing to let the addict know if they see any current, potential relapse warning signs.

Managing lapses and relapses. Recovering alcoholics need to prepare to intervene early in the process in order to prevent a lapse from becoming a relapse, or stopping a relapse before it gets out of hand. The alcoholic's initial response to a lapse largely determines whether there is a return to recovery or movement further down the road to a full blown relapse. Alcoholics may feel angry, depressed, guilty or shameful following a lapse or relapse. They may think I'm a failure, I'm incapable of changing, I just can't do it, or why even bother trying, and these attitudes can fuel the relapse further. Learning to challenge such negative thoughts and rehearsing a plan to interrupt a lapse or relapse ahead of time can prepare alcoholics to take action rather than passively accept that there is nothing they can do.

Lifestyle balance. Recovering individuals can benefit from strategies that reduce stress, improve coping ability, or improve health. These include exercise, meditation, focusing on spirituality, or focusing on achieving a better balance between obligations in life (shoulds) and desires (wants).

(continued on page 198)

Breaking Point
Tiffany Williams

The flying Barbie hits my left shoulder and bounces off, striking my bedroom wall with a dull clunk. I stare at the ceiling as I lie on my bed and begin the process of dissociating; a buzzing starts in my head and the contents of my room fade to a tingling gray. My mother's voice cuts its way through the gauzy veil of my primary defense mechanism in jagged pieces.

"Take all…money…you're worthless…"

A wad of cash rains down to cover my bedspread and me. I finger a dollar bill. A loud crash cuts through my personal barrier, startling me into a sitting position. Eyes wide and glassy, I survey my bedroom through the gray haze. My mother must have slammed the door on her way out; it takes forever to reach that simple conclusion.

The threat is gone and I can focus again, all senses intent on escape. It's the classic fight or flight response, ten minutes too late. I scramble for the essentials: my knife and my spiked wristband. I wrench my window open and slip through it. My feet hit the ground. I'm off and running to my personal haven. I am halfway down my street before the power of external sensation returns to me and I realize that I've forgotten my shoes; the rough gravel of the road's shoulder tears the soles of my feet. But I can't stop now, so I ignore the dull, throbbing pain. I trot down the steep slope of the cement spillway, nearly slipping as the bits of gravel come loose from my feet.

I crouch down on my haunches like a defensive animal, poised on the slope, and release a scream that sears my lungs. The scream develops into a howl of fury and frustration and hatred. Soon I begin shouting obscenities at my mother as though she can hear me. As though she would care.

"I hope you die! *You're* the stupid one! You're the one who's worthless! I hate you, you disgusting, drunken monster!"

I go on and on, often repeating the same words over and over until I'm crying, gulping in huge breaths of air and then letting them out in screams. I'm soon hysterical, sobbing wildly, and then letting out loud, maniacal laughs.

Much time goes by before I can wipe my face free of tears and stand up. A terrifying numbness enters my mind as I begin the walk home. My legs have become numb too, and I step gingerly the entire way, my feet and calves bleeding. I approach my house. All is quiet. Climbing through my waist-high window proves to be a difficult feat. I haul myself over the ledge, aching legs and all. My room is untouched. I gather up all the money my mom threw at me and place it on my nightstand.

It's impossible to rationally express hurt feelings and anger to a woman who is drunk five nights a week. How do I tell my mom "I feel angry," when she's staring blearily at a point somewhere over my forehead, swaying from side to side, unaware? How do I say "My feelings are hurt when you call me worthless," when she's got that malicious glint in her eye and an open can of beer clutched in her hand? I can't—not when I sicken every time I look at her, not when I can't keep the sneer of superiority off my face.

My mother deigns to drive me to school the next morning, but she isn't speaking to me. She's hung over; it's easy to tell. Last night's slurred words sling themselves at me all over again, and I turn my face to look out the window. "Have a good day," I mutter as I leave the car. Stone-faced, she doesn't reply. Even my half-hearted, semi-sincere attempts at reconciliation are ignored. I take one last glance at her haggard, blotchy face, and smirk.

The day slips quietly by in a blur of classes and unrecognized faces. Halfway through fourth period, I receive a text message from my mom. I grimace as I check its contents under my desk. "I'm sorry about last night. Do you forgive me?" I bite my lip, angry all over again. How can she...? But there's no other option. "Of course I do," I text her back, hating myself for playing along with her sick game of emotional torture. The school day is almost over; it's nearly time to go home, and I can feel the nagging dread of being there with her well up in me, as it does every day.

I drag myself to the bus and hope to miss it so I can catch the next one, to give myself another half hour away from home. Ever since she lost her job in October her drinking has gotten worse, to the point where she starts just after she drops me off at school. There's no peace anymore; it used to be that when I got home, I had an hour's respite before she arrived, already tipsy.

It's later that night, when I am soaking in the bathtub to avoid speaking to my now-awake and now-plastered mother, that I receive a shock. My little brother Matthew begins pounding on the bathroom door, shouting incoherently at me. I wrap a towel around my dripping body and crack open the door. I look down at his terrified, pale face, and pray to all the powers I don't believe in that my mom didn't die of alcohol poisoning out there on the living room floor.

"The cops are here," he whispers, urgent.

I drop my towel and slip on a pair of jeans. It seems to take forever to put clothes on my still-damp body. I thrust on my glasses and take that first cautious step out of the bathroom. Matthew is lingering in the kitchen, tears streaming down his face. I enter the living room, and three pairs of eyes settle on me. My mom stares blearily at me, hazel eyes glazed over by a film of alcohol. The other pairs belong to two tall figures in blue: the police.

"They're taking me to the hospital," my mom murmurs, dropping her gaze to the floor.

"Why?" I ask, not understanding why tonight is any different from last night, or the night before that, or for any night in the last sixteen years, as a matter of fact.

"I'm tired of this," she says, and she sounds so defeated. The police are apparently muttering comforting words to us, but they sail over my head. All I can hear is my mom whispering "Take care of Matt," as she is guided out the door. I follow, standing on the threshold. I watch them lead my stumbling mother out to their cruiser and lock her in the back seat. I close the front door so I can't see them pull away and lean against it and let out a sigh.

"Hey Matt!" I call, and he patters into the living room. I stare down at him, feeling bitter. He's making a heroic effort to wipe the tears from his face and seems stronger than he should have to be at the tender age of nine.

"Yeah?"

"What the hell just happened?" I ask, and he lets a panicked chuckle escape before he answers.

"Mom called the cops on herself," he tells me, flopping down on the couch.

"And why is that, exactly?"

"Because she's drunk," he concludes, as if that explains all of this. I shrug, figuring she'll be back tomorrow and that nothing will have changed, except that we'll have a hospital bill on top of everything else that we can't afford.

Despite all the emotions raging beneath the surface, I plaster a smile on my face so that I can present some sort of normalcy in the face of the bizarre. Even though I'm only sixteen, I have to suck it up and spend the night being strong for my little brother. I sit with him and patiently help him with his homework, then read to him from one of his favorite books.

In the morning, I somehow manage to send him off to school on the bus without argument and to go to school myself. It's an even longer day than usual, and I feel the exhaustion seeping into my muscles. This afternoon, I'm too distracted to even bother doing homework on the bus as I usually do. I return home to find Matthew and my mom, sober, waiting for me.

"We're going to Grandma's," Mom says. "Please get ready to go." She seems cautious and nervous, like I'm the time bomb that's ticking away. I drop my backpack in the hallway and shrug.

"I'm ready," I tell her, wondering if she's going to dump Matthew and me off at Grandma's house and go on a drinking binge. Much to my surprise, when we arrive there is what seems to be a delegation waiting for us. My grandmother is there, of course, as well as my mother's brother Kevin, his wife Nancy, and my dad John, who has come all the way over from his town a hundred miles away to be a part of this. We all settle into the living room. An awkward silence descends over our group, and I wonder exactly what is going on. It's not too long before the answer is provided: this family meeting is what amounts to an intervention, called by my mother herself. The topic at hand: rehab.

Hours pass as my family converses around me. I don't offer my opinion until someone asks; I want as little to do with this as possible. Will it be good for my mom? Maybe. I guess I just can't help being bitter anymore. A local rehab center is chosen and called; my mother finds that she can get in for free. The family makes plans to care for Matthew and me.

Dusk is falling as my mom, dad, brother, and I pile into my mom's station wagon and begin the strained drive to the rehabilitation center in the next town over. My dad tries to give a pep talk in his typical irritating, patronizing manner, but I can't reply, even to tell him off. My throat is too stuffed full of cotton to speak.

We walk with Mom to the office and stand staring around in silence while she fills out registration forms. I leave to get a breath of fresh air; I'm getting the pressurized feeling in my chest that means I'm about to cry. As convinced as I am that I hate her, this monster who poses as my mom, I can't help but feel a twist of anguish as I hug her goodbye in the office, with the jaded eye of the attendant aimed at us. It'll take a long while for me to realize that the monster who poses as my mom is *not* my mom. It's the alcohol.

Tiffany Williams is a twenty-year-old college student living in California, where she actively adores cats, music and the English language. Her mother is now enjoying her fourth year of sobriety.

The Journey to Hope
Uma Girish

I closed the door softly behind myself and hastened in the direction of the bus stop. The sky was indigo, the birds getting their last moments of sleep before they awakened to perform the dawn chorus. Flinching from the sharp wind, I huddled deeper into my frayed jacket. The wind and the cold made me think of my mother, father, brother and three sisters. I saw Ma's vacant eyes, my sisters' tears, and my brother shuffling a pack of cards all day long. All three looked to me to fill Father's shoes: shoes he had cast off as too uncomfortable. The previous night he had staggered home at midnight, vodka-sodden. The slur in his speech caused me to make my decision. Now was the time for me. Now was the time to break the chains, before it was too late. So I called my friend Nina and said, "I'll take it. I'll take the job."

Nina and the others thought I was taking it for the pocket money. How could I tell them the money wouldn't go towards shoes and bags and clothes? I was taking the job so I could pay my college tuition and keep my siblings in school.

The street lamps cast a watery light, their strength dimming as a grey dawn filtered through. I craned my neck. No sign of the bus. I glanced at the *salwar kameez* I wore, faded and ready for the cast-off pile. Good enough to wear to a new job? I would be doing the arrival and departure announcements on television at the local train station and would only be seen on train station platforms. But it was the best I had. If I needed more, I could cut up a few of Ma's old saris.

The bus roared up, shattering my thoughts. I picked a window seat, settled my bag in my lap, and thought back to how life had charted the twists and turns to bring me to this place. Eighteen years old and off to my first job as television announcer at the railway station. A picture formed in my head: a row of empty liquor bottles on a kitchen shelf; the thick stack of rupee notes from payday morning that had dwindled by evening.

The fight had gone out of Ma a long time ago. It showed in her slumped shoulders, dark ringed eyes, and the corners of her mouth that succumbed to gravity. She wrung her hands and stared, fear and nervousness competing on her face. My brother stared up at me. My sisters stared up at me. Big Sis was the fixer, a title I didn't exactly want. They believed I had all the answers. They believed I held the pieces in my hand and that I only had to slot them in the right places and the happy picture would be whole.

Why didn't Ma walk out on this man, who was squeezing her dry emotionally and physically? Why couldn't she stand up for herself, get a job and support us? It was so unfair that our lives had to be tied to his, because she lacked the courage to throw her clothes in a suitcase and slam the front door behind her. Resentment and rage boiled inside my chest. The other girls in college all had it so good. The biggest calamity in their lives was being unable to afford the right earring. They would show off their shoes and bags and trade notes on which mascara and lipstick stayed on the longest while I blinked away the tears and smiled even as my heart squeezed inside my chest. Why did it have to be this way for me? All my thoughts and anxieties converged on one person: Father. When would he get home tonight? Would he be drunk? Will we have to call the neighbor to pull him out of the car? Would Ma have to call the Club, the local bars and his colleagues to search him out? My thoughts were constantly filled with shame and humiliation.

On days when a lecturer was on a leave of absence, we were allowed to leave college during those free hours. When the free time was announced the girls whooped and sprinted out the college gates. They made plans to go get coffee, to shop at the mall, or catch a matinee. I stayed in the college library and made notes, read, or simply pretended to look busy. My mind wandered far away as I worried about whether there would be a scene at home that night. I hated to leave college a minute earlier than I had to. It was a haven of sorts. Home was filled with terrors and secrets that embarrassed me. Ma would start her routine lament the moment I stepped through the front door. I couldn't bear it, but bear it I did. I always clenched my jaw and allowed her sob stories to wash over me.

The bus wheels slipped into a rut and jolted me back to the present. Almost daylight. The train station was two stops away. I sat up straight, smoothed a hand over my clothes and rearranged my features. It was time to wear my "outside world" look. Looking pleasant was part of the job definition, even though essentially all I would be doing was parrot the same stale information:

287 Charminar Express from Madras is expected to arrive on platform number 3 at 7.15 am; or, Blue Mountain Express from Kodaikanal expected to arrive at 6.30 am is delayed by 2 hours; or, Mangalore-Secunderabad Special scheduled to depart at 10am is delayed by 25 minutes...

The bus halted, and the ticket collector yelled, "Secunderabad Station!" The stench of urine and fresh cow dung hit me in waves as I got off. I pinched my nose and quickened my pace, picking my way through people sleeping on thin sheets on the station floor, stray dogs sniffing for scraps, and beggars who held out cupped palms, their eyes and hair wild with deprivation. Up a flight of stairs I went, and entered the second room on the right.

Bridget's welcoming smile was like a breath of fresh air. I gulped gratefully. "We have ten minutes," she said, glancing at the Rolex on her wrist. She handed me a typed schedule of train numbers and timings. "Okay, listen," she said, "Tina should be here any minute. She'll do the Telugu announcements, I'll handle Hindi and you do English, yeah?"

Over the next hour I made friends with the camera, learned to take my cues, and tried to look as pleasant as possible. But the early hour and the tensions at home were telling on me. As excited as I was to be on camera, starting my new job, last night's drama kept playing in my head. Ma had shaken me awake past midnight, worried because my father hadn't come home.

"Don't waste your sleep on that man," I'd told her. "Just go to sleep."

"Shall I call Uncle John?" she persisted.

"Call whoever you like ... just don't bother me." I snuggled deeper into my bed.

But now that I was awake I wouldn't be able to shut out what followed. I heard her making a few calls, her agitation fueled when she failed to locate Father. I also heard her tiptoeing to my sister's bed and shaking her awake. It was nothing new. I would lie there, night after night, as the same scene occurred. The car would finally come home, its headlights throwing dancing shadows on our bedroom walls. The engine would hum outside the garage, the car door would slam. The shuffle of footsteps as he would get out and realize that the engine was still running. The car would slide back; the engine would rev louder, the car would lurch forward. When he finally made it to the house Father would sprawl on the sofa, arms and legs splayed like a rag doll. Then Ma would try to revive him by feeding him buttermilk, most of which dribbled down his chin. This nightly ritual bothered me no end. Why did Ma have to put up with this? But she felt she had to. She had never worked a day outside the kitchen in her life. That tied her to Father and all his misdemeanors. Walking out simply wasn't an option.

I love her. I hate her. I love her. I hate her. I hate her more than I love her. No, I love her more than I hate her. The words pounded through my brain. Ma's sheer helplessness, her refusing to free us all from this miserable life, her preoccupation with Father's whereabouts—it depressed me. It also made me determined to grow up to be unlike her. I felt stuck in this life. It was like living in an airless room, and I had suffocated long enough.

But now I must smile because I am on camera, and the world mustn't see my sadness and shame.

One evening soon thereafter, my first pay from the train station job arrived. I ran with the envelope to my bedroom, vibrating with excitement. I threw myself on the bed and drew out the crisp rupee notes from the envelope and fingered them one by one. Six hundred rupees felt like a king's ransom. Just touching those notes spread a warm glow of satisfaction through me. Here it was. Proof that I could do something useful, and be paid for it. I'd broken free of the shackles. In my mind's eye blue skies stretched ahead, and sunshine and the smell of freedom was in the air. That moment, I felt a new me emerge from within. The promise to be everything I could be was still inside me. Father and his drinking could never take that away. I smiled, tucked the envelope under my pillow, and for the first time in years slept a dreamless sleep.

The author's father has remained sober for twenty years now. In that period, he has devoted all his spare time to suffering alcoholics—drawing them into the A.A. fold, by telling them his story of despair and then finding the light, and encouraging them to understand that a better life is possible without alcohol. Wives and children of suffering alcoholics are grateful for his inspiration and guidance and treat him like a Messiah. He has become a leader of sorts in his A.A. group and went on to become the Resident

Director of a detoxification centre. It was his way of thanking God for a new life; the second chance that he had been granted.

Uma Girish is an award-winning writer based in Chennai, India. Her work has appeared in *Christian Science Monitor*, *Women's eNews*, *Massage Magazine*, *India Currents*, *Good Housekeeping*, *Gurlz*, *Imagine Magazine* and *The New Writer*, among others. Uma conducts creative writing workshops at local schools and bookstores and is also passionate about the subject of reading to children—another area where she conducts workshops for both parents and children.

Part VI

The answers aren't "out there"—they are in our hearts...
I have achieved complete membership in the human family...
I tend to believe it to be a **miracle**.

Do You Know the Way to A.A.?
Diane Saarinen

My drinking had gotten out of control and my therapist suggested I try Alcoholics Anonymous. I was ready. And since it was Christmas time, I thought it would make a good New Year's resolution that I could start on a bit early.

I got information from the A.A. website, and when the time came I gathered all my courage and went out on a bitter cold day to attend my first meeting at a nearby synagogue, not knowing what to expect. I arrived at a synagogue that was undergoing construction, scaffolding covering its façade, and no one in sight. I looked to see if anyone had posted any signs about the meeting, but saw none. So I went home, dejected, and continued what had become my daily habit of drinking.

I made a second try a week later. That Saturday morning I went to a church not far from the synagogue. But instead of a meeting, all I encountered was a man in jeans and a flannel shirt selling Vermont-grown Christmas trees in front of the building. I thought for a few seconds, coughed and asked him, "Is this where they have the A.A. meetings?" So much for anonymity. I was surprised by his reply: "Well, I know they used to have meetings here," he said. "I sleep in the church at night rather than drive back to Vermont every day, and last year I used to have coffee in the mornings with the A.A. people. They were real nice." After I looked around a bit more, I concluded there was no meeting being held there that day. But I was closer! At least I'd found a place where an A.A. meeting had occurred. I went home and continued to drink.

For the next foray a week and a half later, I didn't bother with Internet research. This time I telephoned A.A. and was directed to a church a little farther away from my neighborhood. I was very excited. Surely I would find a meeting! But again… nothing! The janitor directed me to the upstairs offices where I was told that if I came back on Wednesday might I would find a meeting. *But I'm ready now*, I thought. *If I go home and wait a few days I'll just keep drinking.*

I had just one hope left: that maybe, just maybe, I was in the wrong church. On my way out I noticed a man outside holding a beer can covered in a brown paper bag. I figured this guy had to know where the meetings were being held! And bless him, he told me I was indeed at the wrong church. I would find the meeting on the next block.

I eagerly followed his instructions and made my way down the street, around the corner to the basement of the other church. People were filing into an assembly room and arranging folding chairs in a circle. I followed suit, as if I had been doing this all my life. I had finally arrived at a meeting! And that was how I at last found my way to A.A.

Diane Saarinen is a freelance writer whose work frequently appears in the *New World Finn* journal, *Finlandia Weekly* newspaper, and on the *Quiet Mountain: New Feminist Essays* website. She is also the book reviewer for *NewAgeJournal.com*. She lives in Brooklyn, New York with her husband, Peter, and their two cats.

My Dark Nights of the Soul
Ruth Fishel

"Every flower must grow through dirt."

— Anonymous

Sometimes we experience an inner calling so insistently that we must listen to it. It might appear as a voice, or a dream, or as some kind of sign. It might come to us as an inner knowing, the simple knowledge that it is time for change, to follow another path. Perhaps we feel directed to a change we don't want to make. It can be so strong that, no matter how painful it might be to make this change, we feel we have no choice: a calling to a new career, a change of lifestyle, letting go of a relationship. A friend once told me he heard it as a wave rolling over him, urging him to come along, come along, come along, until he had no choice but to follow. Responding to the message to serve God, he left everything he had and everyone he knew and joined a monastery. In the end, when he surrendered to the call, he was very content with his decision. My own soul-searching, my struggle for self-understanding, independence and purpose, sometimes appeared to me as a loud, confident "Yes!", other times as a very weak, meek "No", and once as a roaring "Stop!"

I was born in Boston and named Ruth Lois Haase after my grandmother on my mother's side. Because there was already a Ruth Haase, a cousin, in my family, my parents decided to call me Lois, so there wouldn't be any confusion. My father's job took our family to Detroit, Michigan when I was two and a half years old. A few years after our move, the Second World War broke out. For the duration of the war we could get only a one-year lease when we rented a house; we had to move at the end of each lease because the soldiers coming home from the war received first priority for housing. We moved at least four times from the time I was in kindergarten through the fourth grade.

My memories of my life in Detroit are very happy ones. I was a tomboy and loved to climb trees and play ball. There were lots of children in our neighborhood and there was always something to do. Looking back, I remember my confidence and unself-consciousness: I joined all the neighborhood children putting on shows for our parents in our back yards, dancing and singing songs. It was a very carefree time for me.

My father lost his job when I turned ten. My family decided to return to Boston and I left all of my friends behind in Detroit. We moved three more times to three different towns in Massachusetts during my fifth grade year as my father changed jobs. I attended three different schools that year and a fourth one for the sixth grade. As a result, my confidence went underground for many years. I became very shy and self-conscious. It became very difficult for me to make new friends.

We moved, finally, to Brookline, Massachusetts, a town that was at that time home to well-to-do Jewish families. My father, however, had not been able to find a job that was right for him since leaving Detroit. Finally, my uncle got him a very low-paying job in the stock room of a shoe factory. Since we had very little money, we had to rent the second floor of a two-family house in a neighborhood of single-family homes owned by people who were far better off financially than we were. I remember my mother's excitement when she was able to buy six new school dresses for me for $1.00 each at a bargain store in downtown Boston.

I always felt inferior to the other students in Brookline. We walked the two miles to school in those days and I would pass by homes that had bowling alleys in their basements and Cadillacs in their driveways. My father couldn't afford a car until I was almost seventeen; many of the Brookline girls had been given their own cars when they turned sixteen. It's no wonder that growing up I felt insecure, inferior, and "not as good as." But as soon as I found alcohol, I relaxed and felt "as good as." I felt as pretty as, as smart as, everyone else. By the end of my senior year in college I was a daily drinker.

I started a greeting card company while in college and continued to build it after I graduated. I married one year after graduation. I continued my daily drinking but I became sneaky about it. I would pour one glass of scotch while making supper, going often into the kitchen to "check how it was coming along" while actually refilling my glass so it looked like I was only having one drink. Dinner was often very late in those days!

My husband and I had three children. He soon joined me in the greeting card business and it grew. My drinking continued and increased. I was up to almost a fifth a day. In the back of my mind I thought, "I can stop whenever I want," but I knew I was lying to myself. I tried. For the last five years of my drinking I tried. I would wake up each morning and promise myself I wouldn't drink that day. But I would leave work and my car, as if it had a mind of its own, and would pull into a different package store each day (if I went into the same one, day after day, the clerk might think I had a drinking problem!).

Somewhere deep inside me, my soul was screaming for help. I heard "Stop!" over and over again in my mind but I couldn't. Towards the end of my drinking, I would buy just a pint in the afternoon and promise myself I would only have one drink from it.

When the pint was empty my resolve was empty as well and I would rush out to the package store before it closed to buy another. Once home, I would drink until I passed out, wake up in the middle of the night and finish whatever was left in my glass because, as my daily mantra went, "I'm not going to drink tomorrow."

But I had arrived at a place in my life where I hated myself so much so that I could not continue to live the way I was living. I thought I was the worst mother, the worst wife, the worst daughter in the entire world. While I dearly loved my children, somewhere inside of me I always felt that I was meant to do more. But I had no understanding of what the "more" could be. I always had a yearning, a craving, as if something was missing and I had no idea where to find it. This emptiness and longing has been described by others as spiritual deprivation. We feel a longing, a craving, and we try to satisfy it with everything from alcohol and drugs, to food and sex, to gambling and thrills, only to find that while we might feel better temporarily, the emptiness always returns.

During the years of my alcoholism, I struggled trying to understand and know God, questioning whether there even was a God and desperately seeking meaning and purpose in my life. While in college, I gave up struggling with the question of the existence of God. After much soul-searching, I became an agnostic, comfortable with the conclusion that maybe there is or maybe there isn't a God. It was clear to me that one could never know for sure and if some people wanted to believe there is a God, that's fine for them. I didn't need to believe. I was strong. I could handle anything.

Years later, alcohol proved me wrong. I could not handle everything. I could not stop drinking. We had a nice home, a boat and two cars. On the surface, everything looked fine. But deep inside I knew it wasn't fine. I no longer just *wanted* to drink every day: I *had* to drink, every day.

I became more and more depressed; I finally hit a bottom. In deep anguish, I opened myself to the gift of desperation and joined a recovery program. I began going to self-help groups whose members had gone through what I had experienced, people who couldn't stop drinking but were able to turn their lives around. They were loving, supportive and full of joy. They gave me their telephone numbers and asked me to call, telling me that by helping me they were helping themselves, that was how they stayed sober. I began to discover what I had to do to become free of all the unhappiness, self-pity, self-consciousness and shame I carried deep within me. A new way of life began to unfold. I was just twelve steps away from a light heart and a new purpose in my life.

The program suggested that I ask for help from a Power greater than myself. By now, I was finally desperate enough to take the advice of people who had suffered as I had suffered, but had learned to stop drinking. I was ready to try anything, even though I still didn't believe in God. I prayed, "If there is a God you will understand and if there isn't, it doesn't matter, but please keep me away from a drink and a pill and a desire for a drink and a pill."

Psychotherapist and author Marion Woodward writes, "...at the very point of vulnerability is where the surrender takes place—that is where the god enters. The god comes through the wound." That's exactly the way it happened for me. The miracle happened! I was able to go through a day without a drink; and then two; and then ten. For a while, I would still pick up a drink after ten days or three weeks, but the days between drinks increased over time and I began to feel a bit better. And finally, after many long months, I lost my desire to drink and I have not had a drink since.

I came to believe in this power greater than myself, this God. I knew on my own I could not stop drinking. Something greater than I was working. Early in my journey to God, someone suggested that I put an extra "O" in the word God and to consider God a power for good and love. That made sense to me and I still, thirty years later, believe that. God does not always come in the form that we can recognize. God spoke to me through the people who were in recovery, people who knew my pain, despair and hopelessness, because they had been there.

Dr. Gerald May writes: "Our incompleteness is the empty side of our longing for God and for love. It is what draws us towards God and each other." When I finally did pray to this God that I did not believe in, relief came, and soon my desire to stop drinking was miraculously lifted. It was enough to prove to me that I was not God. Years of pain and struggle gradually ended and I had a spiritual awakening.

Over the following years I searched in many directions to find my joy and purpose. I learned and practiced transcendental meditation until I discovered mindfulness, another form of meditation, which I practice to this day. I learned about herbs and crystals, self-hypnosis and labyrinths. I even made a labyrinth in my backyard. I read about Buddhism, Kabbalism, Christianity and Judaism. I discovered there are many paths to spirituality. I looked into Reiki and became a Reiki 2 Practitioner. I had my palm, stars and Tarot cards read. While putting on spiritual retreats for women in Sedona, I went to the seven energy centers. I studied books and tapes, wrote books and made tapes, went to retreats and workshops and facilitated retreats and conferences.

All this time I was learning. It was a process. I was clearing my mind of all old, misguided concepts, letting go of negative judgments about myself and others and opening my heart to invite God in to my life. Over time I learned the truth. The answers aren't "out there"; they are in our hearts, just where the Creator put them.

Ruth Fishel, M.Ed. is a nationally known author and meditation teacher whose books include the best-selling classic *Time for Joy*, *Living Light as a Feather*, and *Change Almost Anything in 21 Days*. Ruth is co-director of Spirithaven and has helped thousands of people feel better about themselves spiritually, mentally and physically. She can be reached at spirithaven@spirithaven.com or through www.spirithaven.com.

A Simple Cup of Coffee
Lucy Brummett

I was raped by my alcoholic brother when I was five years old. Soon after, my alcoholic father walked out on our large family, leaving us to be raised by a neurotic mother. Verbally and physically abusive, she was unfit to raise her children. I could not bear watching my siblings be hurt, so when I was nine years old I made the decision to be a mother to them myself.

We were a poor Latino family who often went hungry. Sometimes we had to go barefoot to school. After my father left, my mother got pregnant again and gave birth to another little girl, Laura. She didn't love this baby, and told me she was going to sell her. I threatened to call child services. She said that if I wanted her to keep the baby, I would be responsible for her care. From then on, wherever I went, Laura went, too. People sometimes say I was robbed of my childhood. I have to agree.

When I turned sixteen, I married a man nine years my senior and soon had three girls of my own. Their father turned out to be as bad as my father. Unable to deal with still more abuse, I turned to alcohol for relief. I began going to Catholic Bible study classes because I was always offered some wine at the end. When I would return home tipsy, my sister would be infuriated with me.

My husband grew intolerant of my drinking, and I finally left him after eighteen years of marriage. It tore my heart to leave my girls behind but I had to get out of there, and I never intended to leave my girls forever. I went to Chicago to be with my sister for a while. What was supposed to be only a two-week separation turned permanent instead. My husband met another woman and any chance of reconciliation was shattered.

After this, my alcoholism nearly destroyed me. I drank night and day. Every weekend I would go to a nightclub and listen to a band. Some nights, I would leave with one of the band members. It felt good to get some attention, and I would accept beer after beer.

One night, while in a car with a musician, I glanced behind me and could see the bright city lights fading into the distance. I started to get scared. I'll never know if my drink had been drugged, but I remember blacking out and then waking up to a hand covering my mouth tightly. Then I lost consciousness again.

The following morning, I woke up in a motel room in wrenching pain. I got up to look outside; I didn't know where I was. A cleaning lady was just outside my door. When I opened it, she got scared and led me back to my room to wash my beaten face with a warm washcloth. It was then I realized that I had been raped. He had violated me, stolen my wallet and left me to fend for myself. The cleaning lady wanted me to call the police, but I refused. Who would believe me? I was the one who had been drinking, and I had left with him of my own free will. This kind woman only had twenty dollars to her name, but she gave them to me with directions to get back home. I'll never forget her kindness and generosity.

Two buses, a train and three blocks on foot got me back to my sister's apartment. When she saw me she was frantic and wanted to take me to the hospital. But my breath still smelled of alcohol and I refused. I told her I had been in a car accident. She didn't believe my story, but she backed me up when she told my brother-in-law what had happened. I never told her the truth.

This should have stopped anyone from drinking, but I only drank more to help numb the pain of the memory. Finally, one November day in 2002, I got into a car when I was drunk, with the intention of killing myself. But things didn't turn out the way I had planned. Instead, I think God took my hand that night. He led me to Alcoholics Anonymous.

The group consisted of Latino men who were all speaking Spanish. As I sat down, I remember being terribly afraid of them. A man approached me and asked what I wanted to drink. I thought of alcohol, and I asked what he had. He said, "We have coffee, pop, tea or water." A simple cup of coffee saved my life that night. I listened to all of them tell their stories, but I was too embarrassed to tell my own. When they asked who was there for the first time I slowly raised my hand.

It has been four years since I joined that group. It has done so much for me. Ever since, I feel better about myself. I have learned to deal with my problems without drinking. I told my story to that first group of men, and now I go to other Latino Alcoholics Anonymous groups and tell them as well. I feel happiest when I can help women who don't know A.A. is the answer.

God is the primary being, and He is the one that did it for me. Second is Alcoholics Anonymous, and third is myself. When my sister died, I had the willpower to stay away from alcohol because I knew that it wasn't the answer to my grieving.

While I might not have the power to change the events in my past, I can help dictate my future. Life is a precious gift that I will never again take for granted, and being able to share that with my daughters and grandchildren is priceless.

Lucy Brummett is a freelance writer with a weekly newspaper column on a variety of topics. She resides in Fremont, Ohio with her husband and their two sons. Future books in the making include a bilingual children's picture book and an inspirational book for women who want to change their current career path.

(continued from page 172)

Does Treatment Work?

There is a considerable body of scientific evidence demonstrating that treatment for alcohol use disorders is effective. One major study of alcoholics found that at one year followup, alcoholic clients reduced the percentage of drinking days per month from 80% to 20%, and reduced the average number of drinks per drinking day from 17 to 3. Many studies show greater reductions of HIV rates among treated clients compared to those who do not receive treatment. Treated individuals use less medical services after treatment and report better mood than untreated individuals, and many show increases in rates of employment as a result of treatment.

(continued on page 227)

Reprieve from Insanity
Peter Wright

I grew up in an impoverished Irish Catholic family in Liverpool, England. There were four of us, five if you count God. My mother told us that He was forever with us, but He was someone I didn't understand or like. He was invisible, but always present. He was powerful but never gave us anything. And we had to worship Him at mass every Sunday and give Him money. This view of my Maker stayed with me—until I needed Him.

My father was a marine engineer and spent most of his life at sea. I hardly ever saw him. He never spoke of God. He was killed in a marine disaster in 1937 when I was ten. My mother suffered greatly at his loss. I didn't. I didn't know him.

Sure that she and the rest of the family would be granted entry into heaven if there were a priest in the family, my mother arranged for me to attend a Dominican boarding school, with the hopes that I would become the family's celestial passport. During the seven years I spent at that school, one of the priests made some nasty moves on me which curdled any positive thoughts I may have harbored about the priesthood and further damaged my image of God. I chose, instead, to go to sea like my father.

Life at sea for this seventeen-year-old apprentice was no picnic. Reserved and painfully shy, I didn't fit in with the other boisterous lads. Nevertheless, I wanted what they had, and found it one evening off the West Coast of Africa:

"Try this, Peter. It'll put hair on your chest"

I took the proffered gourd of African gin, overcame its dreadful smell and drank. I became a real sailor in no time. I had discovered the secret of "being one of the boys." Two days later I got drunk at the next port—the gene connection had been made and my future mapped.

I stayed at sea for the next twenty-three years, passed the required examinations and became master of a transatlantic freighter. But somewhere between that first revealing drink in West Africa and my last desperate gulp in a desolate apartment in Portland, Oregon, I had crossed the line between social drinking and alcoholic binging. The final transition went by me unnoticed but not to those around me. "Better do something about your drinking," they cautiously advised. I told them that I drank no more than any other seafarer and that I certainly was not alcoholic. They simply didn't understand me.

In 1965 I left my wife and five children in England for another woman who lived in San Francisco. I lied to both women. Convinced that I would be able to control my drinking in the U.S.A, I rationalized that my move would solve my problem and benefit everyone. I had a good job. I sent money to England. What more could I do? Completely unaware of the trap I had just set for myself, it never occurred to me that alcohol, and alcohol alone, had deprived me of reason. I now had two nemeses: guilt and my disease.

After a short period of overwhelming anxiety, my drinking escalated. My days began at dawn with Scotch whisky. Two-hour luncheons broke the days' back, and I passed my evenings sneaking drinks I had hidden all over the house.

Eventually my significant partner insisted I enter a recovery program. I reluctantly agreed but denied that I was alcoholic. I just needed time to cope with my stressful job. Set in the wine country in the Napa Valley, my twenty-eight days went by effortlessly. Meetings of Alcoholics Anonymous were daily ingredients, features of which I didn't understand. I often heard simple phrases such as *One day at a time*, *Easy does it*, and *First things first*. What did they all mean? I concluded that the purpose of this program was to teach me a lesson on moderation—to drink like a gentleman. It would be another thirteen years before I took my last drink.

In spite of my pretensions, I didn't drink for a few weeks after I left the rehab. I felt better in every way and my relationships improved. It was no surprise to me though, when the thought came to me one evening on the way home from work: *I'd better celebrate*. Within ten days, the disease had resumed its hold over me. I hadn't listened to the lectures on its progression. I found myself like a sailor heading for shoal water with neither rudder nor compass.

On January 26 1976, the managing director fired me. Unreliable, he had said. Feelings of fear and indignation stopped me dead in my tracks. I took a cautious look at myself. I knew that I often drank a little too much, but why fire me? I could control my drinking—if they had told me to. Denial that I had a serious problem was forever uppermost in my mind. I would show them.

Two weeks later I started my own marine investigation business. I stayed off the liquor and business thrived. I didn't know, however, that just below my shiny surface the disease lay dormant, waiting. I didn't know that I was addicted to alcohol, that I was alcoholic. And because my mind was infected with the disease, I had a frontal lobe Rationalization Committee in session, all the time persuading me that I didn't really have a problem and that I could drink without any serious consequences. The essence of my committee's philosophy was simply, *If things are going well, celebrate with a drink; if things are not going well, comfort yourself with a drink.*

One evening after nine months of enormous success, I thought that it would be nice to have a glass of wine. After all, there is hardly any alcohol in that stuff. A week later my business folded and once again I became enmeshed in the labyrinth of insanity. The Rationalization Committee's job was done.

For two years I went from job to job, eking out stipends from various groups who remembered me from the old days: *Got to give good old Peter a job!* One group sent me to North Africa. *Go easy on the booze, old boy; if you get drunk in Algeria they'll lock you up and throw away the key.* For the next eighteen months, during which I traveled back and forth, I lived on Antibes in Africa and Johnny Walker in the U.S.A. My last benefactor sent me to Fiji to inaugurate a new service. I had been dry for three weeks. Inevitably, I fell in with an old shipmate and arrived back in San Francisco a week later without remembering the event. My significant partner refused me entry into the house.

I had nowhere to live and hardly a brain to work with. Searching for a place to sleep, I went home. My partner called the sheriff and I got my night's sleep—in jail. This happened on several occasions. A judge finally sentenced me to three years probation in a halfway house.

Then a miracle happened. Friends Charlie and Noreen, in whose debt I shall forever be, took me to the city detox on Howard Street. They told the counselor to take care of me. But I wasn't ready for a miracle, so I walked out looking for drink.

Full of some Thunderbird donated by some of San Francisco's forgotten, I ended the night exhausted, spiritless and contemplating suicide while crouching beneath the freeway. It was March 7, 1978, my youngest daughter's birthday. Rambling thoughts drifted through my brain. *How would my mother have reacted to my plight? A drink would see me right. Where do I go now?*

The following morning, dregs of my sanity led me back to the detox I had left the evening before. After a twenty-eight-day program I was admitted to The Oliver House, a halfway house on Ninth Street, San Francisco. Several weeks of listening and learning from people with my disease dulled the edge of my pride. I learned that love also existed beyond the bedroom and caring meant one drunk looking after another drunk. I made friends and settled in. We were all obliged to attend daily meetings of Alcoholics Anonymous. I heard the words but failed to make the connection with God.

Rusty, the house manager, influenced my early recovery in an unexpected manner. She knew I was having difficulty with the program and took opportunities to chat with me in her office. Her life story, and the honesty with which she told it, chilled me. I began to take a hard look at myself and discovered that being honest with myself, just as Rusty had been honest when she talked about her life, was a very frightening experience. Without complete honesty, not only in recovery but in all parts of my life, I would never have achieved sobriety.

One afternoon Rusty handed me a book, and suggested I might like it. The moment I read the title, *The Hound of Heaven*, I was taken back to my childhood days. I had seen my mother reading an elegantly bound copy of Francis Thompson's epic work, and asked her why she was weeping. She hugged me and softly said, "It's about a poor man looking for God."

The opening stanza goes like this:

I fled Him down the nights and down the Days;
I fled Him down the arches of the Years;
I fled Him down the labyrinthine ways of my own mind
And in the midst of tears, hid from Him.

Thompson's opening statement emotionally stopped me in my tracks. I researched Thompson's life. Born into a devout Roman Catholic family, he had been selected by his father for the priesthood and sent to Upshaw College. The Proctors at Upshaw had sent him home, saying that he wasn't suitable material. He entered the literary field and joined a group of writers in bohemian London where opium, the latest fad, was said to open one's mind. Francis became chronically addicted. With recovery on his mind, he composed this epic confession.

The discovery of this amazingly honest piece of literature was the first glimmer of the dawn of my understanding of spirituality. I was able to piece together the messages I heard from Alcoholics Anonymous, Rusty's honesty and the cries for help so heartbreakingly presented by Thompson.

Almost a year had passed in the comparative comfort and safety of The Oliver House. I became healthy again and even had started a course on alcohol counseling at the University of California at Berkeley, but I had become complacent. A friend of mine in the steamship business told me about a job opening as superintendent on the Columbia River, Oregon. Whatever spirituality I had absorbed vanished overnight. Whatever peace I had accumulated in my troubled mind, I forfeited. I was cured. I wanted out.

Rusty was heartbroken. "You are doing well, Peter, but you're not ready." Her last words to me as I got in a taxi outside The Oliver House were, "You know where to find us."

That winter in Southern Oregon was the coldest on record. The river froze and shipping traffic was limited. I had a lot of time on my hands. My tiny apartment in Portland became a dismal cell within a week. I attended A.A. meetings but it wasn't the same. I tried to make women friends, but that didn't work either. Work picked up when the ice broke and my days and nights became stressfully intense. I stopped going to meetings.

On my way to Everett one icy morning, my radiator hose blew. Exiting down a steep off-ramp, I skidded to a halt outside a tavern. A red neon COLD BEER sign invited me in. My committee, which I had been successfully ignoring, told me it was a sign that

I couldn't ignore. The effect of alcohol was immediate. I felt on top of the world again but my elation was tinged with foreboding. Suppose they were right about the progression of the disease?

They were! My committee had done its job well. Ten days later, I was almost dysfunctional. Holed up in my cavern, I questioned my sanity. It was beyond my comprehension how I could have once again reached this state of utter debilitation. I was terrified by my frantic attempts to make the nightmare go away by drinking until it had no further effect.

Crocuses were peeping through the snow on the morning I crept out of my apartment and headed for the airport. Rusty greeted me, but not kindly. Another treatment program! Would I ever get the knack of getting and staying sober? What was I missing? I lay in the gutter of life.

One of the counselors at Starting Point, Owen, called me into his office one morning.

"It's a long time since I met anyone like you, Peter. You are reasonably bright but you lack the milk of humanity. You are a selfish snob. You are, it appears, the only person in your life."

How dare he talk to me like that? But it worked.

Following a twenty-eight-day program at St. Joseph's Hospital in San Francisco, I entered Serenity House in the city. The stricter rules in this halfway house gave me the impetus to become a spiritual self-starter. After a grace period of eight weeks, we were obliged to go out and work to pay the rent. Mandatory periods of quiet time gave me the opportunity to think. I was able, finally, to connect Thompson's humility and honesty with the program of Alcoholics Anonymous. I surrendered to a higher power that, I finally came to believe, would restore me to sanity. I also looked inside myself, and found parts of a power that I call spirituality.

The more I read (and heard) Thompson's cries for help, the better I knew that I was on the right road. People in Alcoholics Anonymous who had sailed these perilous waters before me, and who had charted the reefs and rocks, told me that they had rarely seen a person fail who had carefully followed their suggestions. They knew me. They know of my disease.

This time, it worked.

After three years of actually living *one day at a time*, the honeymoon was over and the work of true recovery began. I began clearing up the wreckage of my past. My children were foremost in my mind; they had suffered without understanding. Not without anger and often painful emotion, we drew closer. Today I am happy to tell you that I have an international family, five children in England and two in the United States, who love me and have taken this drunken sailor back, not as wreckage but as a father paying loving dues. With the help of my family and my friends at A.A. I've managed to stay with it. I recently held my twenty-third dry birthday at an A.A. Roundup. These occasions never fail to bring tears to my eyes: tears of gratitude to my wife and friends who have tolerated me, but more especially to the fellowship of Alcoholics Anonymous. I learned of the promises made to me by those who knew from experience the rewards of sobriety. They were so right. I'm living those rewards every day.

Born in England in 1926, Peter Wright was educated at a Dominican boarding school where his mother hoped that he would become a priest and, eventually, the first English Pope. Instead, he went to sea in 1943 as a midshipman in the Merchant Navy, rising to the rank of Captain. Peter had his last drink on January 30, 1983 and since then has had a successful career as a marine investigator.

Desperation
Kim Mallin

"It's a stomach virus," I told the E.R. doc as I clutched my stomach, racked with pains after two days of vomiting. I wondered, *does he believe me?* Did he know that this "stomach virus" actually came in bottles of cheap red wine? I'm pretty sure I wouldn't have believed it. I'd seen people like me before, drunks staggering in and hollowly disguising their complaint as something else. Yes, I'd seen plenty of people like me: when I was in residency. I was a doctor, and on that dreadful Christmas of 1995 I was also a hopeless alcoholic.

If I close my eyes, I can still feel the sting of sleet hitting my face as I walked out of the emergency room on that Christmas, taste the bitterness in my mouth, remember the waves of nausea rolling through my stomach. I walked towards the cab that one of the hospital staff had been nice enough to call for me; I had no one to pick me up.

This was not how I'd planned to spend Christmas. My parents lived two hours away and my brother, sister and I were planning to celebrate the holiday with them. I hadn't told them yet that I had lost my job earlier that week. I hadn't told them yet that I was drinking again, but it wouldn't be long until they figured it out. This wasn't the first time we had been through this.

I remember walking out of that E.R., embarrassed, swearing to myself that I would never drink again. I got into the cab and gave the driver my address. All I had was a hundred-dollar bill, and I asked the driver if she could break it. When she said no, I asked her to look for a convenience store, hoping we could find one open on Christmas morning. I walked into the first open store we saw, and walked out with three bottles of wine.

How had I gotten to this miserable place? This place where I couldn't even trust myself to go into a store without buying some type of alcohol? I wasn't some bum living under a bridge. I was a good person: I had graduated *magna cum laude* from college, in the top third of my medical school, a practicing physician. So how did it come to this? It happened one drink and one pill at a time, around the time my dad declared himself an alcoholic and started attending twelve-step programs. I never thought of him as an alcoholic. I knew he drank beer almost nightly and that it made my mom angry, but he was never arrested, never hit anyone or lost his job. I thought he just drank to relax.

After experiencing a few blackouts in my early twenties, I decided to be careful about my drinking, a decision reinforced when I learned in medical school that alcoholism is a genetic disease. I was usually able to control my alcohol use. But I was completely unprepared for the euphoric release of my first painkiller, taken innocently enough for a headache. Within six months, I was busted for prescription forgery. And that was just the first time.

I spent the next three years in and out of treatment centers. After I was arrested the second time, I lost my much-prized surgery residency, only five months before graduation. The day I "resigned," one of the professors in my surgery department spoke to me, trying to understand why I couldn't seem to stop my drinking and drug use. He finally shook his head and said, "You must either want to go to jail, or you must really be an addict." I remember being puzzled about my obvious need to go to jail: I couldn't fathom being an addict.

I lost my medical license, twice. I got divorced. I made the newspapers, twice. The first time was for charges made against me for "prescription writing for my relatives." The article discussed my fraud while describing me in court as looking "demure in a peach and white striped dress." The second time I was not viewed as demure. The headline on the story about my second case described me as "Convicted Felon."

I wish I could say that following that court case I got clean and sober and stayed that way. I can't. Recognizing my addiction for what it was and accepting it proved extremely difficult for me. I fought my addiction with everything I had. Those years in and out of treatment centers were not easy ones. I learned about desperation, failure, inadequacies, and fear. I became a master manipulator and liar—anything to allow me to keep getting my booze and drugs, no matter the cost. I switched from pills to alcohol when I lost the ability to write prescriptions. I couldn't imagine my life without drugs or alcohol.

I called my parents that Christmas, after getting home from the E.R., and telling them that I wouldn't be coming home for the holiday. That I was having a little problem with drinking again, but that I would get it under control. They offered to come get me, but I refused. Thank God they didn't come rescue me. I desperately needed to reach my bottom. Slowly I was losing my life...and myself.

I spent the next few days in a haze. Every day I woke up, or came to, thinking, *Today I'm not going to drink. Last night was the last time.* I would go to a twelve-step meeting, pick up a white chip to show my desire to stop drinking, and be drunk within a few hours of leaving the meeting. I remember during that time a friend calling me, begging me to get help, saying that he skimmed the obituaries daily, fearing that he would see my name.

On the third morning following my trip to the E.R., my attempt at sleep was disturbed by an annoying muttering. No matter how tightly I held the pillows over my head, I couldn't escape the noise. Assuming it to be the radio, I reached over to turn it off. But the radio wasn't on. Confused, I staggered out of bed and went into the living room, thinking I must have left the TV on. But I hadn't.

I raced through my apartment, looking for the source of the noise. I remember suddenly stopping, leaning against the wall and slowly sliding down to the floor as the truth dawned on me. As inconceivable as it seemed, the only answer was that the noise was coming from inside my head. *I was hearing things.* Auditory hallucinations. The significance of this hit me hard.

I threw on some clothes and ran out the door. I was terrified. I jumped in the car and headed for the house of a woman I knew from a twelve-step meeting. I remembered she had talked about hearing voices, too. Maybe she could help me. And she did.

That was my last drunken Christmas. As horrible and painful as it was, it was the beginning of a new life for me. I didn't get sober and stay sober just then, but it really was the beginning of the end of my drunken days. But it was a hard beginning. The following April I was kicked out of the third treatment facility I had been in since asking for help. I kept being kicked out because I would sneak out and drink while in treatment. I remember standing outside of Wayside House with nowhere to go. I had no job and no medical license. I couldn't go home to my parents: I had broken my probation by drinking and leaving the state without permission so there was the possibility of going directly to jail if I went back to North Carolina.

Something happened for me that day. I tend to believe it to be a miracle, because nothing else had ever been able to stop me from drinking and drugging my life away. My counselor suggested that I move into a local halfway house, so I did. I put aside any dreams of being a doctor and focused on surviving a day at a time without using drugs or alcohol. I committed to staying in the halfway house for six months and to following its rules.

Graduating from the Lighthouse felt as significant as graduating from college or medical school. I spent another three years working as a library assistant and staying active in twelve-step programs. I came to understand and believe that I was an alcoholic and an addict and always would be. I stayed connected with the Professional Recovery Network (PRN) in Florida and they continued to monitor me throughout this time. They helped keep alive the possibility of my return to medicine. Tough as they were, I wouldn't change those years. Those hard-earned lessons have proven invaluable for my personal and professional growth. I wouldn't have the strength I have today if it weren't for those struggles and those successes. With the encouragement of the PRN, after three years I did eventually decide to try to get back into medicine. I had a whole new set of survival mechanisms and a stronger ability to empathize. I understood emotional pain and, better yet, I had learned how to walk through it. I knew what it was like to have a chronic illness. Surely, these were experiences that could only make me a better physician.

Every year around the holidays, I get a little melancholy as I think about the past, but I have such gratitude for the life I have today. Not all gifts come in pretty packages, tied up with big colorful bows. Sometimes they don't even look like gifts; sometimes they can look like the worst thing that could possibly happen, and it is only with the passage of time that the gift becomes apparent. So Christmas of 1995 was my worst—but it helped point me in the direction I needed to go. I now have a wonderful husband, a great job, a loving family. My work schedule is filled with patients who trust me to take care of them and their families. I could go on and on, listing the material gifts I've received, not to mention the immeasurable gifts, such as increased self-esteem, improved spirituality, and actually liking what I see when I look in the mirror. Life is great. And I know I wouldn't have any of it if I had not been given the gift of desperation on that cold, lonely Christmas so many years ago.

Born in the mountains of North Carolina, Kim Mallin is a graduate of the University of North Carolina-Wilmington and the East Carolina University School of Medicine. After four years in a General Surgery residency, she took several years out of medicine for recovery reasons, working in plant nurseries, bookstores and libraries in South Florida. Missing the "true South" and the practice of medicine, she returned to the Carolinas in 1999, attending the Medical University of South Carolina to complete a Family Medicine residency. She is a regular contributor to *Sasee* and *The Daniel Island News*, and has had several articles published in *Medical Economics* and *Running Times*. She now practices family medicine outside of Charleston, South Carolina.

Do As I Say, Not As I Do
Ed Lamp, Ph.D.

There are times when it seems like only yesterday that I was young and still living at home. In reality it has been over fifty years. We were a normal family and seemed to be like most others in the Twin Cities. Alcohol was some part of life for almost everyone who lived there. There were some people who didn't drink, but they were a minority. Those of us too young to drink knew that our parents usually drank, but we didn't think much about it.

My dad was one of those. He would have a drink every night when he got home from work and more than a few beers on a weekend. Since he never became aggressive or physically abusive to anyone, we accepted it rather than make waves. For whatever reason we were taught to believe that serious alcohol-related problems didn't happen in our society. Our image of a "real" alcoholic was someone who was very rich and living it up by drinking to extreme, or someone like a bum living in the slums with a six-pack in hand. Being middle class meant we were both above and below those sorts of drinking problems.

The older we got, the more oblivious we were to what was going on around us. Looking back now, I realize that this was most likely our way of protecting ourselves from reality. I did notice, however, that Dad always worked hard on house-related projects all weekend. I can still hear him telling us, "This is the only way things get done." Always along with this work came more than a bottle of beer or a drink or two of the hard stuff. It was obvious that the harder he worked the more he drank. The alcohol was like a pick-me-up, or a painkiller. My father's work was always of great quantity and quality, so we didn't pay much attention to the drinking.

By the time I entered high school, the hard work on weekends had greatly increased, as had the drinking, and it was starting to affect his behavior. Finally, the time came when we could see the toll it was taking on him. His speech was becoming slurred and every night, right after dinner, he immediately went to sleep. His family and their social lives were both suffering a slow but steady decline. I am sure my mother knew that something had to be done, but back then the idea of a middle-class alcoholic wasn't talked about or even considered. I imagine that there were other families on our block with similar alcohol-related problems, but the big secret prevailed. Not even the closest of friends talked about it amongst themselves. In fact, our secret was so tightly guarded that my sister and I never talked about it with each other. And you can bet your last dime that my mother, who held the family together, never mentioned it. Back then people believed that if you kept your job, went to church and paid the bills, everything was okay.

Sometimes my classmates and I would get together and share stories that we were forbidden to talk about with our families. Stories about who had drunk what last weekend were usually our favorite part of those conversations. Frequently, it was a classmate, relative, or someone else we were supposed to see as a role model.

Adults would usually tell us, "Do as I say, not as I do." Here were our parents, teachers, and church leaders—our supposed role models—telling us that drinking to excess was not good for us, when most of them were heavy drinkers themselves. This was very difficult for us to understand, because the people we saw drinking seemed to enjoy it. Their unintended message was that if you wanted to enjoy life, you drank; it was the social thing to do.

Dad continued to drink too much, but by then we were off to college and didn't see much of it. Mother continued to do what wives have done for too many years: she pretended it wasn't happening. Then one day, in a strange way, the problem solved itself. My father, by then seventy-five, contracted a serious skin disorder. The best doctors couldn't figure out the cause. One doctor prescribed a drug that nearly killed him. Finally, when he was near the bottom, almost dead, he made a bargain with God: he would never drink again if he could go on living. He lived, and never did drink again, not even to toast his 50th wedding anniversary.

I do not believe that God stopped him from drinking or cured him of the itching. At best, I believe that God stood by him and supported the strength that he had all along. Needless to say, Dad's abstinence made all who loved him happier.

Looking back over my life, I can see some positives that might be the result of my father's drinking. I graduated from college with a degree in psychology and have taught a class on alcohol and health most of my adult life. I know my understanding of alcohol abuse and its effect on drinkers' lives has made me a much better teacher. I know that living with Dad made me more determined to use my knowledge and compassion to help others live better lives. Although Dad drank to excess, he never directly harmed anyone other than himself. I have no doubt that his obsessive drinking taught me to never abuse alcohol, and to help others to do the same.

Ed Lamp holds a Ph.D. in health and has both taken and taught college courses dealing with alcoholism. This work has provided him with a "real life" source of information that brings the classroom into reality.

Blessed by Truth
Hannah Smith

It was 10:30 on a hot August night at Grand Lake when I heard the scrape of metal porch furniture and slurred cursing. I had come inside from the patio to get away from the huge mosquitoes and the tension of waiting for Dad to get back from his predawn fishing trip. We were all afraid he might have drowned, but no one would say it. So I sat under a fan and escaped into my novel.

My stomach tightened as the screen door banged open and Dad stumbled into the family room of our cabin. Bill, only fourteen but already almost the same height as Dad, carried him. I sat, riveted, as I watched Bill heave the dirty two-hundred-pound body, stinking of sweat, fish and alcohol, onto the bed in the next room. Dad was snoring the moment he was on his back. Bill took off Dad's wet shoes and set them on the floor. We exchanged looks of sorrow mixed with relief as he came out of the bedroom. "I found him passed out on the path to the dock," he said softly. Then he left to sit outside with Mom, trying to hold the family together one more night. I was four years older than Bill, and it had always been my job to keep my parents from divorcing. I fought back tears to see my little brother now taking on the job.

We knew Dad's drinking kept us from solving the problem that had trapped our family. Yet the problem didn't have a name. We would think he had quit for months at a time, and then just as we were beginning to trust him again, the old patterns would return—so many times I can't count. We could not fathom why he did this when he was so good at everything else in life. An executive in the booming oil business, he had the respect of his employees and bosses. As I grew older, I heard stories of the hard drinking they all did together in the early days in the field. It apparently went with the business. Neither set of my grandparents drank so I couldn't make sense of it. As a little girl I felt sorry for my father, angry, confused, and, worst of all, ashamed. "He drinks," we would whisper to people when forced to explain his behavior.

When Dad was dying, we sat in his hospital room for days, listening to the death rattle get louder. More than forty people, our whole extended family, lined the walls of his room when he died. We were all relieved when he finally gave it up. His death left a big vacuum where the daily task of dealing with him had once been.

It wasn't until after he died that I actually called him an alcoholic. And I didn't even realize that what had killed him had a name—cirrhosis of the liver. Shortly after his death, as I was chatting about him with my neighbor, she mentioned that her father was also an alcoholic. I was stunned to hear her use the term. Maybe I had never even said that word. She began to talk about her family, and I realized she was giving words to the silence and shadows of my past. It felt jarring, and I knew I had not escaped, as hard as I had tried. It was a part of me, and I felt swallowed up by it, knowing bad things were still ahead.

It wasn't until the wrenching pain I felt a few years later, when my husband left, that I sought help. When he began to have professional success, he seemed to come apart, wanting to be free—"I think I can be happier," he said. I was devastated. I felt as helpless as I had as a child when I couldn't fix the problems that were tearing us apart.

He didn't drink and neither did I, but without my being aware of it, we had been falling into the patterns of an alcoholic marriage, patterns that had filled my childhood home. One day I was describing him to another friend who had drinkers in her family and what she said stopped my heart. "He sounds like a dry drunk. That's a drinker who has stopped drinking but hasn't worked on his pain from the past," she explained. "Dry drunks are often controlling and angry without their coping drug, and worse to live with than a drinking drunk. He sounds exactly like that." Her words hit a raw nerve and I knew that the flaw was inside me too. Having absorbed that knowledge, I decided to accompany her to the next Al Anon meeting.

I had a typical first timer's reaction to the meeting. I felt I was in the wrong place. But I probably sensed the Lord for the first time at this point, knowing He was preparing me for what followed. I wanted to run but knew there was no place to go.

It was 1980 and the Adult Children of Alcoholics (ACOA) movement was just beginning, with Melody Beattie's book, *Codependent No More*, just off the press. About ten of us started a small group in a church basement, and the serious healing began. The first task was to create a safe environment, free from criticism of others. We learned never to give our opinion of someone else's story, except to say that it reminded us of one of our own. We limited our comments to our own personal issues and experiences. The second was to understand that it is our responsibility to take care of ourselves. After saying the famous twelve steps every morning, we needed to say the word HALT (which means Hungry, Angry, Lonely, Tired), as a kind of status check, to be repeated any time we became aware that we were under stress, times when we were most likely to fall into destructive thinking patterns. We learned to recognize the onset and consciously divert our actions towards something healthier.

As we learned to trust one another, we began to describe our own damaged places and take responsibility. We massaged away the spiritual numbness that causes denial and celebrated each new truth and strength. When we were together, we could take the really scary stuff out into the light where we weren't alone with it. It bubbled up a little at a time as we were ready to deal with it. We were developing a map to mark the way out of the choking despair that surrounds an isolated soul.

The group grew to several hundred people from all social strata, meeting in many places, one every night of the week. The most valued gatherings were those held on holidays, when "normal" people are having their warm, loving celebrations at home, leaving the rest of us to emotionally hemorrhage for slow, suffocating hours. The group gave each of us the opportunity to grow up—to go back to the memories of growing up in alcoholic households—memories that had warped our maturation and stunted our emotional growth. Through gentle but honest openness from others, we could see our errors and hear our own stories told through people in the room who might appear very different from us on the outside. The role of each of our own family members was played out as we talked on the selected topic of the night. Compassion, understanding and strength began to replace confusion, panic and helplessness.

I had always loved my father but I began to cherish him. I became able to see beyond his flaws through adult eyes and respect his achievements, and his love for us and the courage it took to face his pain every day as he provided for us. The people in the meetings began to reflect a depth of understanding and love that was beyond human capacity. I felt the Holy Spirit many times as years of anger and sorrow fell away, replaced by gratitude, repentance and joy.

Then the real miracle began to happen. I could see that the pain was a tool to break through my self-centeredness. Without it, I would have persisted in trying to live a life of shallow happiness instead of seeing struggle as the only path to a life of deeper meaning. Through the blessing of my past scholarship, I began to see evidence of this in history, literature and religion. It connected me to the generations before—even to mankind, and set me on a new course of study.

No longer do I live life on the outside trying to get in, but now I feel that I have achieved complete membership in the human family. And I know I'm not only loved and blessed by God, but have a responsibility to tell my precious story—to demonstrate the beauty and celebration of life rather than remaining stuck in the pain of the past. And to let others know that one can only answer the questions asked, not give endless sermons on the subject. The saying "when the student is ready, the teacher appears" is well understood in the groups. I will pray that all those who read this are ready for the teacher.

Hannah Smith grew up in the Midwest in an alcoholic home where there was no physical, sexual or verbal abuse and knows how rare that is. Her home had much love but, like the others, had a deep sense of helplessness and a lot of sadness. She has a professional background in commercial real estate and small business development and has been a writer for five years.

Till Death Do We Part
Katrina Hunt

Alcoholism is a disease with enormous power. Like a terrible storm, my husband's addiction to alcohol left a path of destruction, threatening to destroy our family and marriage. As I fought to keep my family together and save my marriage, I came to understand that I could not fight it alone; I needed help to win.

We married when we were eighteen. A year later our daughter was born. It was another thirteen years before we had our second child. From the beginning, our married life was a struggle, since we were both so young and financially unprepared. But at the same time, we both felt that we were ready for the responsibility. As I looked forward to the role of wife and mother, I had no idea I would find myself taking on another role as the wife of an alcoholic.

I knew my husband had a problem with alcohol when his drinking became more than just occasional. I would tell him my concerns; he would tell me it wasn't a problem. Because I so wanted to believe him, I tried to ignore the drinking and pretended everything was all right. I hoped he would get better. I was trying to keep things at home as normal as possible for our children, hiding what was going on from my family and friends, ashamed and embarrassed for anyone to know. Besides, it was difficult explaining to anyone what was wrong when I didn't understand the problem myself.

As his drinking progressed, my caring and loving husband, this wonderful father became a different person. We began to argue about everything and nothing I did was good enough for him. I tried to be the perfect wife and mother, cooking his favorite meals, keeping a spotless home while working full time. I thought this would make a difference, and that things would get better. I didn't understand that he couldn't see what his drinking was doing to us.

Eventually, my husband did seek help through Alcoholics Anonymous and he stopped drinking. He thought he could stay sober on his own and stopped attending meetings. Just when I thought alcohol would no longer be part of our lives, my worst fears were realized. After two years of sobriety, he started drinking again. I was devastated.

He tried to convince me that he could control his drinking. He promised that things would be different. I thought of my wedding vows, my promise to stay with him in sickness and in health. I loved my husband, and as bad as it was for me, leaving him was something I could not do when he needed me most. I wanted us to be a family so badly that I believed that, somehow, it would work out.

The years that followed were terribly difficult as the effects of the disease began to resurface. His addiction to alcohol began to take total control of our lives and his guilt turned into anger towards me. He blamed me for everything that had gone wrong. It wasn't long before I believed that I was at fault for his drinking and I began to doubt every decision I made. Soon my life had become unmanageable; even the simplest things felt like difficult tasks to accomplish.

But just when I felt I couldn't handle any more, a tragedy changed everything. My mother died, and four months later my father had a stroke that left him paralyzed. My life seemed to falling apart and I felt that there was nothing I could do about it. My father's passing less than two years later made me realize that I had no one but myself to depend on. I knew that if my life was going to change, I had to change. I couldn't control life, but I could control how I let it affect me.

So I accepted the fact that my husband was an alcoholic and that it was a disease. I had lived my life around my husband's drinking, doing everything he asked just to avoid arguments. If he was having a good or bad day, so was I. Every decision was based on how he might react. While my husband lost control of his life, I realized that the one thing he did have control over was me. I learned to accept what couldn't be changed, and I starting changing the things I could. I was able to slowly let go of the past and start living for the future. I knew how much my husband loved us. I wanted him back. I realized my battle wasn't with my husband's drinking, it was with the disease of alcoholism. I knew little about this disease, but I knew the pain it caused. I realized that if I continued to make excuses and solve his problems, he would never see the damage that had been done.

My husband had always been very close to our children, and I was grateful for that. But as she grew older, our teenage daughter became disappointed and distant, which was hard for him to accept. She began spending time with her friends, leaving me feeling lonely and wondering how I would make it through. My youngest girl then became the joy of my life. Knowing how much she needed me, I found the strength and the courage to keep going.

The more control over my life I was able to take back, the more I noticed positive changes in myself and in the children. I stopped reacting to my husband's behavior the way he expected me to. I learned to say what I thought without arguing. My husband was speechless at times, as he could see he no longer controlled me. I started doing the things that made *me* happy, and I learned to laugh again, at times at my husband's foibles. I realized that laughter was part of my healing and it helped me to cope.

Eventually my children and I became a family, spending time together and enjoying life without my husband. He could see what he was missing and I knew he wanted to be part of it. It was hard watching him hit bottom, and at times I felt sorry for him. He became depressed and withdrew from everyone. I wanted to help him, but I knew he was going to have to help himself first. He was tired of living his life that way and finally admitted he was powerless to control his addiction. When he made the decision to accept help, our road to recovery began.

But it was truly a long and painful journey. I was sure he had never noticed all I had been through and sacrificed. Then one day I found a letter he left for me. He wrote, "I am sorry for all that I put you through. You deserve better. You are a good mother and wife, and I am glad you stayed with me. Please hang in there with me, I will make things right. I love you, your sober husband."

I couldn't stop crying, and at that moment I knew in my heart that all I had been through was worth it. Today he has found his sobriety. He attends an A.A. meeting every day and has become involved as a member. I have a better understanding of this disease through Al-Anon and the meetings I attend with him. We are now a family recovering from the effects of this disease. My husband and our daughters are close again and he realizes he has a second chance to be a father to both of them. I have my husband back, and our married love continues to grow daily. Beyond any doubts we know the meaning of "for better or worse" and "in sickness and in health." And there isn't a doubt in my heart that we will be together, as we promised so long ago, until "death do we part."

A professional in the medical field for nine years and an aspiring freelance writer, Katrina Hunt resides in Alabama with her husband of twenty years and their two children. She shares her story in the hope that it will encourage those coping with this disease.

(continued from page 198)

Where Do We Go From Here?

AUDs are associated with many problems and increased rates of mortality. However, many effective behavioral therapies and medications exist to help individuals with AUDs and their families. A variety of professional services and mutual support programs such as A.A. are available to address alcoholism. It is clear from outcome studies that there are substantial benefits to treatment even though the path to recovery is not always smooth.

The alcoholic who engages in a long-term recovery process increases the chances of stopping drinking and making positive lifestyle changes. Since alcoholism is a disease that affects the family as well as the alcoholics, families can benefit from professional treatment as well as mutual support programs like Al-Anon. Such involvement enables family members to support the alcoholic's recovery and reduce their own emotional burden and deal with the problems caused or worsened by the impact of alcoholism on the family system. Professionals can help by identifying alcohol problems and facilitating help for the alcoholic as well as family members. Viewing alcoholism as a treatable disease with effective medications, therapies and self-help support programs such as AA is critical. This must be based on an attitude of hope.

Dennis C. Daley, Ph.D. is Professor of Psychiatry and Chief of Addiction Medicine Services (AMS) at Western Psychiatric Institute and Clinic (WPIC) of the University of Pittsburgh Medical Center in Pittsburgh, Pennsylvania. WPIC is one of the leading psychiatric institutions in the country, and is internationally known for research in the basic sciences and clinical care. Dr. Daley has been involved in developing and managing treatment services for addiction and dual disorders for nearly 30 years. He has developed models of clinical care in the areas of relapse prevention, dual disorders, group treatment and motivational therapy. Dr. Daley continues to provide therapy to addicted patients.

He has authored over 260 publications including books, book chapters, recovery guides, journal articles and educational films on dual disorders, recovery, relapse prevention, and family issues. He has written treatment and counseling manuals for clinicians on mental illness, addiction, relapse prevention, cocaine addiction, treatment adherence, family treatment, and group counseling. Dr. Daley has been or is currently a Principal Investigator, Co-Principal Investigator, Investigator, consultant or trainer on many research studies sponsored by the National Institute on Drug Abuse (NIDA) and National Institute on Alcohol Abuse and Alcoholism related to treatment of individuals with alcoholism, cocaine addiction, other substance disorders, depression, bipolar illness or other psychiatric disorders. He is currently Principle Investigator of the Appalachian Tri-State Node of NIDA's Clinical Trials Network project, which is comprised of research centers and community treatment programs throughout the U.S.

Antoine Douaihy, M.D., is Associate Professor of Psychiatry and Medical Director of Addiction Medicine Services (AMS) and the WPIC Inpatient Dual Diagnosis Unit at the University of Pittsburgh School Of Medicine. He provides medical leadership for AMS, which treats over 8,000 patients annually in more than 20 programs. Dr Douaihy is a practicing psychiatrist and lecturer on substance use disorders and HIV psychiatry. His research and publications focus on dual diagnosis/patient recovery guides and HIV psychiatry. Dr Douaihy is an investigator in numerous NIDA and NIAAA clinical research projects on substance use disorders and dual diagnosis and was recently included in Best Doctors in America 2005-2006. He and Dr. Daley have collaborated on clinical programs, research, and teaching for the past 8 years. They also have co-authored many chapters, books and recovery guides for patients on issues related to addiction, or addiction combined with psychiatric illness.

Better than Better
Leslie C. Lewis

When my daughter was born I came to understand the kind of love that the Prophets speak about. This kind of love reconstructs our identity at the cellular level. This love is difficult to distinguish from pain, and leaves one gasping for breath under waves of emotionality. I came to understand how a heart could melt, become fearless in its desire to protect the innocent, and vulnerable to sentimentality. I became a dazed and happy initiate into the Society of Mothers.

I also became my mother's peer, able to converse with her in a new language. Mutual motherhood has given us a way to relate to each other that releases me from being an imperfect reflection of Daughter and naturally bestows upon my mother the deserved stature of one who has gone before me. Our mutual challenge throughout the years of my mother's alcoholism, her recovery, and her current struggle with lung cancer, has been about perceiving and relating to each other as whole people.

Twenty years ago I attended my first Al-Anon and ACOA meetings. I heard the speaker say, "First it gets better, then it gets worse, then it gets different." *What the hell does that mean?*, I thought. I was there for a permanent dose of "better," and hoped that "different" was just a euphemistic way of saying "better than better." As sobriety became the backbone of my mother's life, and recovery became part of mine, I discovered that different is better than better, but not in the way I had initially conceived.

When my mother entered a residential treatment center for alcoholism at the age of 46, she was consuming a fifth of vodka a day in the isolation of suburban Chicago life. From that day forward, she would remain sober through extreme trials of emotional hardship. Just one year into her sobriety, her parents were brutally murdered in their home during a robbery. A few years later the police would forcibly remove my paranoid schizophrenic father from our house as part of a divorce decree. Marrying for a second time, she would spend some of the most contented years of her life with my stepfather in a cozy retreat on a small Michigan lake. But he suffered a stroke and slowly deteriorated over a four-year period until his death at the age of seventy-six.

My mother remains sober today as she undergoes radiation and chemotherapy treatments for lung cancer. My mother believes that if there is a worst possible case scenario, it will probably happen. She frames this outlook as realism, and despairs over her inability to believe in a personal God. Her unbridled anxiety displays itself in relentless insomnia, and her terror of dying a miserable cancer-related death has resulted in depression mercifully abated by antidepressants. She confided to me that this has been one of the only times she has thought about drinking.

The week after she entered rehab, I flew back to Chicago to visit her. The changes in her appearance and demeanor were extraordinary. She was no longer puffy nor was her face red, and her speech was clear and deliberate. She seemed happy and joked about tipping back a few on the morning she was due to arrive at the treatment center. She talked about how, for the first time in her life, she believed that something, some power greater than herself, really cared about her, and had seen to it that she received help at just the time when she could accept it. I squirmed internally at some of these outpourings, having embraced a kind of detached agnosticism that allowed me to practice utter self-reliance (a stoicism that would soon enough see me to my own personal bottom two years later). But this was trifling compared to the relief that seemingly erased years of resentment. I consciously knew my mother as a part-time drunk from the time I was about eleven, although her drinking had begun several years before that. I had spent most of that time in a silent fury over her drunkenness, and now I could stop being furious. At the moment, that was enough.

When I returned to New York a few days later, her rehab counselor requested that I be part of a phone counseling session in which I would talk about the impact my mother's drinking had had on me. I did not want to do this. At the time, ours had been the typical alcoholic family, engulfed in silence and peopled by heroic achievers and supporting enablers. Alone in my apartment, nauseous, awaiting the counselor's phone call, I prepared to reveal wrenching truths that I was sure would destroy her, and possibly me. When the call came, the counselor assured me that this was for my mother's sobriety and would help her. I found this hard to believe, but my mother offered the same words of encouragement. I had lived for so long under the protection and safety of silence that speaking out meant shattering my identity and abandoning myself to possible annihilation.

I blurted out, "It was like having two mothers, a mother that I loved and a mother that I hated. I loved the mother who was sober, and I hated the mother who was drunk!" At that moment, I just desperately wanted to be with the mother that I loved, now sober twenty-four hours a day, and who just might stay with us forever.

Of course, Saint Vicky, the loved mother, was only real in a partial way. For many years after she stopped drinking, I could only relate to my mother from this perspective, a person with a tragic history (her father suffered from bipolar disorder and was addicted to prescription pills and alcohol), miraculous cure, and heroic sobriety. I had no desire to root around in the trough of disgust and resentment formed by her alcoholism. Denial was easier.

After some years, this relatively safe construct crumbled, and those long-buried resentments returned to consciousness and demanded recognition. This was a painful time for my mother and me and, at my request, we didn't speak for two years. I had to learn how to bring Saint and Drunk together and become fully open to the tenderness and injury that inevitably surface in all deep and lengthy relationships.

The drunken mother of my youth was a caricature of female helplessness and maudlin emotionality. While sobriety dissipated the severity of that persona, remnants of her self-pity would occasionally become barbed comments about my lack of support and understanding. But my mother always possessed a core of attributes without which my world would be a barren place. My world would be a barren place without her softness of forgiveness, her appreciation of nature, her artistic and creative talents.

After our two-year hiatus from each other, we began a shaky communication without knowing exactly what to expect. It has not been the same as it was before, and that is good. In fact, it is better than better, because it is based on seeing clearly. We have become two adults in each other's presence (most of the time) and I am often astonished at how different we are while sharing the same biology.

When my mother was first diagnosed with lung cancer, she created a small wall-hanging entitled "Breathing Room," her last piece to date. I am looking forward to seeing it, as artists often communicate more thoroughly in their artwork than in words. I constantly marvel at how her mind freely imagines the world in unique colors and shapes, and translates that vision into cloth, dye and fiber, pulling the viewer in to her stylistic rhapsody of ideas. I fantasized about how she would create a series of cancer-themed works that would become famous, decorating the walls of some hallowed research center or prestigious fund-raising organization.

No, we will stand together, side by side and look at "Breathing Room," the title of which I will take to heart, for that is just what I need to give her on the oftentimes demeaning, occasionally uplifting, and mostly uncomfortable path of being a person with cancer. I will refrain from interpreting and simply ask questions, curious to know who my mother is in this work and in this world, resting in the wonder of three generations of female diamonds coming out of the rough together.

Leslie C. Lewis is the former Executive Director of the Dispute Settlement Center in Norwalk, Connecticut, and has been involved in the field of conflict resolution and mediation for the past eleven years. She has worked as a musician, teacher, information technology consultant, technical writer and corporate project manager. She occasionally broadcasts topical essays for Connecticut Public Radio and currently writes non-fiction articles and essays about family life, conflict and the environment. An avid gardener and herbalist, she brings the green world's rhythms and gifts to her husband, daughter and two stepdaughters.

Drunk

Sara Ekks

"To regret one's own experiences is to arrest one's own development. To deny one's own experiences is to put a lie into the lips of one's own life. It is no less than a denial of the soul."

—Oscar Wilde, De Profundis

I don't remember my first drink and I don't remember my last. I don't remember my first because it was a given, not an exception. In a good European family, you give the kids a half-glass of wine with dinner on special occasions as soon as they can see over the holiday table and hold the cut-glass stem. None of this puritanical American neurosis about alcohol. Besides, everyone knows that wine aids the digestion. Prosit! Sweet-but-tart German white wine is perfect for children. Hey, Kool-Aid! "Serve well-chilled." The bottle is bright green, like 7-Up. If there's an inch or two left of it after dinner, no one's going to notice if I drain it. No coffee allowed until age ten or twelve—it's too harsh for children.

My first drunk was at age ten, with the family, completely supervised and comical, ha ha. My grandfather put cherry brandy in the Shirley Temples. I really enjoyed dancing that evening. My beige pleated skirt levitated up whenever I spun around and the bow fell out of my hair. All the adults laughed, it was so funny. The bar was in the basement "rec room," brown nub industrial carpet, grossly voluptuous couches, goldenrod Formica bar with matching vinyl-seated stools, altar-like television in a dark wooden box, and my favorite, the taxidermified head of a deer on the wall behind the bar, between steins hanging from pegs, Edelweiss in a glass frame, and an Irish prayer about the wind being at your back printed on a linen flag. I passed out on the orange-striped couch. My father carried me to the family car, a Volkswagen station wagon, and put me in the back seat for the drive home.

My first drunk on my own was acquired in the passenger seat of Stephanie's red Chevette on our way to the Hüsker-Dü show at the Arlington Theatre. Steph's theory was that the cops were looking for kids getting trashed in parks, church parking lots, and other secluded areas, but that on the interstate they were only looking for speeders. Hence, one of the safest places to get high was going the speed limit. Her driving was fine, but with the bumps, I still managed to get a lot of vodka on my pants as I tried to pour it into the cans of Sprite. I couldn't drink it straight, yet. She was happy to smoke pot instead, and wasn't too upset by my clumsiness. "Oh, my God," she intoned as we missed our exit, "I am so high. I am so high. I am so high." I nodded in recognition and slugged down my drink, fishing a can of pop from beneath the seat to mix up a fresh one. The next morning I had my first hangover, fortunately at her house, a long, hot, shower and speculation as to why I had such a headache.

My first attempt to dry out was at age nineteen. I lasted three months.

My first realization that perhaps I'd really better kick it, and for good this time, came six years afterwards, through keeping a journal. The record made me consider the possibility that a daily six-pack and a few shots were not reasonable levels of indulgence, even if they were alternated with days of just red wine (the only reasonable thing with Italian food) or antiseptically scented gin and tonics, or vodka, medicinal and efficient, with cranberry juice, if I had a urinary tract infection.

I quit.

My far-from-the-first realization that I had to ditch my boyfriend at the time came from his repeated insistence that I could drink again, "Any time that I wanted," his persistent efforts to buy me the standard beer or the favorite scotch and his inability to accept statements such as, "This decision is very important to me. I need you to respect it." The friendly bartender at Club Shovel, Melvin, who occasionally braids his beard, noticed my switch to soda and asked, "Taking a little time off, with the breakup?"

I replied: "Nope, sobered up," and added, "What am I doing here?" He laughed.

I don't remember my last drink, not because I blacked out, but because I had been taking longer stretches of time off, saving binges for the weekends, counting, attempting other means of limitation and control. I was somewhere in what was to be an experimental length of time out and decided to go permanent. "Enough."

I dried up, but I was still a sick woman, because I thought of myself as permanently banished from the land of alcohol, the beloved country, all those fuzzy drugs, all those miles of labyrinthine walls to shelter myself from actual existence, never again, a plate of glass crystallized in air between me and it, forever in exile from a much-loved kingdom. When I died, I'd be going, I'd be going, to where rivers of whiskey are flowing, and Aidan would sing Irish ballads to me and the gang would, of course, seem much more witty and attractive and convivial than they actually are. Everyone would be charming and festive and raise their glasses when I came to the table. There'd be crisp, clean gin and tonics; rich, tongue-wrapping scotches that have mellowed in wood for decades before burning your gullet; candied little liqueurs; straightforward lakes of beer; and just for me, an infinite bottle of red wine. And I'd sit beneath a tree on a hilltop and watch the setting sun forever, landscape unrolled to show that it's somewhere in Spain. My back would be against the bark of an oak, a blanket between me and the dried grass, and I would drink that sun in a goblet that never emptied, smooth green glass neck sliding under my palm, lifting it to fill the glass and never getting drunk, just buzzed.

But I will not know alcohol again in this life.

I carried a torch for Aidan, my old drinking buddy, throughout my first marriage. We recited twelve-step language to each other getting drunk together. If he was broke, I'd enable him. Funny how rarely the inverse occurred. That summer, when we were both out of work, we'd dedicate the days to drunkenness, walking along the avenue to the liquor warehouse to buy cases of beer with credit cards, hiking back through ninety-degree heat. He'd carry the case; I'd carry the whiskey.

Our celebrated summer afternoons truly started when I cleared off a space on the wooden kidney-shaped front room table and he stashed the case in the fridge—easy to do, because the fridge generally had nothing else in it but a sad orange, a brown banana, three film cartridges, and Lyra's stash of Beck's. Aidan fished the church key out of the kitchen drawer full of forks, spoons, and cutlery, no two pieces the same, and brought it out to the front room, two beers in his left hand held by the necks. I peeled the foil off the whiskey. We settled onto opposite ends of the couch, a sagging trap of repulsive olive hue, eroded threadbare patches on its arms alternating with paisley brocade that grew into algae tentacles and held you down to its battered cushions by sunset. He pried the cap off one beer and handed it to me, then dispensed with the lid of his. I raised it to him in toast and then sucked off the foam that sprang up from the neck. Then we clinked bottles. "Recognition is the first step on the road to recovery!" Aidan announced. I closed my eyes and tilted the bottom of the bottle towards the ceiling. The first sip is the sweetest. It seriously seemed like a wall full of sockets getting the right plugs, switches flipping, flips switching, all systems go into calm, physical gut relief, the assurance that all was right in the world: you had alcohol. Half a bottle in me in one gulp, I could relax and attend to the serious business of shooting the shit and gradually downing the rest.

Coming to on any given day, I alternately dozed and attempted to recollect the events of the tiniest hours, the ones between 1 A.M. and 4 A.M. that can really get you in trouble. I always had premonitions of the blackouts, always knew when they were coming. I'd go to the bathroom to piss or puke or splash water on my face, and when I raised my eyes to my reflection I could wave good-bye to myself, know that I was on the edge of the utter oblivion that I both feared and craved. I gazed at my image in the mirror, a disordered set of smeared features and jumbled parts, cosmetics dripping, lips askew, face in crooked disarray, and smiled as Consciousness, or the Superego, or Ground Control to Major Tom, whispered: "You're gone. We're going. You're gone. Goodbye. Goodbye. Goodbye." Then the effect was like an old movie played for a room full of restive kids on a day too rainy for recess. The sights lost focus, became grainy and streaked, and then an occasional frame of black appeared, and then another, dark squares falling in rapid succession, until finally the film broke and left black blankness and even the clacking of the ancient projector faded from hearing.

Journal entry, February 19, 1995:

> *...I think that it may be time for me to sober up. Is this necessary? I have no doubt that my depression last night was linked to the previous two days' drinking. I drank four or five beers, or was it six? And had a couple of one-hits at Tracey's on Thursday, and then, on Friday,*

split an excellent bottle of a 1991 Cabernet Sauvignon with Abdul, and then I went out with Lynch to the Fireside and had a number of drafts—five, six? And then Jed bought me a shot. Didn't drink yesterday: ran errands—breakfast out and a trip to the pet food store. There was a beautiful big chocolate-colored dog there and an amusing little pug in a sturdy purple harness—as if it could ever break away.

I'll still hang out with my old crowd, but have met many splendid and amazing individuals who also decided to quit drinking. One evening I find myself at a party at Aidan and Naomi's. One useful thing to remember is to feel free to leave. I decide that it's time for me to go. I pat Tracey's shoulder and go get my jacket, waving good-bye to one or two particular partiers, and trip as I step around Donald.

"Sara!" Donald yelps with obvious distress. "Have you been drinking?"

"No, Don," I laugh. "I'm just clumsy."

"Good." Donald's a real sweetheart. His voice is tinged with relief. "I think about quitting sometimes, and when I do, I think of you, that you've done it." I feel like the neighborhood sobriety poster child, and I am no role model. I squat down and put my hand on his knee.

"Well, I'll tell you what, Don," I feel obligated to say something and decide to try the truth. "I can honestly tell you that it's the single best decision that I've made in my life. I'm not saying that anyone here has a bad life, but it's what I needed to do to improve mine, and it has." He nods at me, earnest and reassured, and we say good night.

I grab my navy peacoat from the rack and do inventory for departure. Cigarettes in the left pocket, keys in the right, hat hanging on the hook next to somebody's tan Carhartt canvas jacket.

"Sara." I turn and see Aidan rotated in his seat, elbow braced on the arm of the chair, chin drawn incrementally inward so that he looks up at me from beneath an overhang of brow ridge. He raises his right hand to chest level and undulates his fingers. "Good-bye."

"Good-bye, Aidan."

"Good-bye, then." He's still waving, still looking up at me. I make my palm flat and spread-fingered and flap my hand sideways like the goofy plastic cut-outs attached to the interior of car windows with suction cups and wires, a competition orange Mickey Mouse glove emblazoned with "Have a Nice Day!" or something, and then stop and pull the stocking cap on, knit covering each ear.

"Good-bye, Aidan. See you."

"Tuesday."

"Right, then."

It's been raining outside and the steps are slick. Despite the rain, the car starts on the first try.

Sara Ekks is the pseudonym of a Chicago writer who has received national literary awards for short fiction. Her prose has appeared in anthologies and her poetry is featured in both academic and experimental publications.

A Look to the Future of Alcoholism Treatment
Ron L. Alterman, M.D.

O God, that men should put an enemy into their mouths to steal away their brains!

—*William Shakespeare,* Othello, Act 2, Scene 3

Like all addictions, alcoholism is viewed by society far differently today than it was even a generation ago. Once considered a "social disease" caused by poor self-control, a weak constitution, or a lack of faith, alcoholism is now viewed as disease like any other—caused by biological mechanisms and potentially treatable, once the underlying pathophysiology is understood.

Contemporary neuropsychiatric research suggests that addiction, whether to narcotics, cocaine, gambling, cigarettes, alcohol, or even chocolate, is associated with specific alterations in brain function that can be studied in laboratory animals or in humans with the help of powerful imaging tools like *positron emission tomography* and *magnetic resonance imaging*. Research indicates that addictive behavior seems to be controlled by a dysfunctional reward system located in a part of the brain that developed long ago known as the *limbic lobe*. When working properly, this reward system causes an organism to remember and return to places where it previously had pleasurable, life-affirming experiences such as eating tasty food or engaging in sexual intercourse. When such resources are scarce, as they were until modern times, this system is beneficial, reinforcing behavior that increases the likelihood of encountering such vital resources in the future. However, in the current age of plenty, where pleasurable commodities such as food are readily available, inexpensive, and craftily packaged and promoted for sale, this reward system can become overwhelmed and maladaptive, creating addiction and causing an individual to eat even when not hungry, smoke cigarettes through a tracheostomy even after his cancerous larynx has been removed, or drink alcohol even after drinking has destroyed the quality of his life.

The transition from casual substance use to addiction can be seen in changes in the chemical substances found in the brain known as *neurotransmitters*, which transmit messages within the brain's reward system. Under normal circumstances, pleasurable experiences such as sexual orgasm, drinking alcohol, or eating highly caloric foods cause the release of the mood elevating neurotransmitters called *dopamine, gamma-amino butyric acid* (GABA), and *endogenous opiates*. These chemicals provide positive reinforcement for these activities by creating a sense of pleasure and cause the organism to seek the resource or perform the act again and again. But, in response to the release of these mood elevators, the body's *homeostatic* mechanisms, which seek to maintain the body's *status quo*, attempt to counterbalance these effects and bring the body back to a state of equilibrium from its pleasurable "high." To do so, the brain increases production of hormones, including *corticotropin releasing factor* (CRF), a so-called stress hormone, while decreasing the levels of other substances such as *neuropeptide Y* (NPY), an *endogenous anxiolytic* (like valium).

Under normal circumstances, such as with the occasional drinker, these homeostatic mechanisms will return the brain to its pre-arousal state. However, if the pleasurable act is repeated before the brain is returned to baseline, and particularly if the activity is repeated a number of times, homeostasis will not be achieved and may be replaced by *allostasis*, a mechanism that seeks neurochemical stability in a rapidly changing or over-stimulated environment, in essence, establishing a new equilibrium level, or set point, within the brain. Allostasis exaggerates the counter-responses to the repeated, mood-elevating stimulation to which the addict subjects his body. Ever larger increases in CRF and decreases in NPY contribute to the hopelessness, irritability, and anxiety that characterize withdrawal symptoms. In addition, changes in the neuroreceptors of the brain through which the abused substance acts reduce the mood-elevating effects of the pleasurable substance, forcing its more frequent use in ever larger doses. Eventually, rather that seeking the desired substance or activity in order to elevate mood, the activity is performed only to avoid the negative symptoms associated with its absence. Ultimately, the pleasure initially associated with the activity is lost, leaving only the pain and unease of its absence.

It remains unclear whether, once homeostasis is disrupted, the addict's brain can ever return to its original set point. Months and even years after quitting their abusive behavior, addicts crave the substance or activity to which they are addicted. Relapse is common, especially if the addict returns to the environment or the relationships associated with the addictive behavior or, as is often the case, if the addiction was caused by an attempt to self-medicate a psychiatric illness such as depression, schizophrenia, or bipolar disease. The average member of Alcoholics Anonymous will tell you that only death cures alcoholism; that he or she is a recovering addict for life.

It is hoped that man's advancing understanding of the pathophysiology of addiction will result in breakthroughs in its treatment and a decrease in the economic burden addiction poses to our society. Medications designed to manipulate the reward system and stem the cravings that result in relapse are under development. Replacement drugs such as methadone and nicotine patches seek to help addicts avert the risky behavior associated with their addiction. Behavioral modification and faith-based initiatives are mainstays of therapy that have proven effective for many.

One promising avenue of research involves a new technology, known as deep brain stimulation (DBS), which may one day alter our approach to treating addiction. DBS involves the insertion of a series of electrodes into specific targets deep within the brain. The electrodes, inserted through one-half inch wide holes in the patient's skull, are connected to an electrical pulse generator, similar to a cardiac pacemaker, which is implanted beneath the skin of the abdomen or chest wall of the patient. The pulse generator delivers electrical stimulation to the deep brain target, modulating the function of those brain cells. The effects of DBS are far-reaching, since neurons in one part of the brain typically influence the activity of neurons in many other parts. As a result, over the last 20 years, DBS has revolutionized the treatment of movement disorders such as Parkinson's disease, essential tremor, and dystonia. Preliminary evidence suggests potential applications of the technology for obsessive-compulsive disorder, epilepsy, Tourette's syndrome and even depression.

Recently, a team of German physicians who were conducting a trial of DBS for patients with severe, medically resistant depression reported on one patient who had suffered with both depression and alcoholism for most of his adult life. He had failed all prior attempts to beat these illnesses and viewed DBS as his last resort. One year after the surgery, the doctors found that the patient's depression was no better; however, without additional treatment, he had spontaneously stopped drinking. Interestingly, the target of stimulation in the brain, known as the *nucleus accumbens*, is part of the limbic lobe reward system. This appears to be the first reported evidence to suggest that DBS may have a positive impact on addictive behavior in humans. As this is just one case, the report must be viewed with tempered, even skeptical enthusiasm. Nevertheless, the outcome is very exciting and presents the possibility that a whole new field of inquiry into addiction and, more importantly, a completely new way to treat alcoholism and other addictions more effectively may soon be upon us.

Dr. Ron L. Alterman is the Director of Functional and Restorative Neurosurgery at Mount Sinai Hospital in New York City. He has held academic positions at New York University School of Medicine (1995-1997), University of Pennsylvania School of Medicine (1997-1998), and Albert Einstein College of Medicine (1998-2004) where he was Assistant Professor of Neurosurgery and a director of stereotactic and functional neurosurgery at Beth Israel Medical Center. Board certified in neurological surgery, Dr. Alterman is well known for his work on deep brain stimulation for Parkinson's disease, torsion dystonia, and tremor. His clinical interests include image-guided surgery for brain tumors and benign spinal disease.

Afterword
Caregiver, Heal Thyself
James Huysman, Psy.D.

About four years ago, Leeza Gibbons and I, the co-founders of the Leeza Gibbons Memory Foundation, were asked to write an article for *Recover Magazine* on why caregivers who are themselves recovering alcoholics were relapsing in greater numbers than other recovering alcoholics and addicts. It is estimated that there are over 50 million caregivers in the United States today, and that number is expected to rise to over 80 million in a decade. If we assume that one in ten people in our culture suffers from the disease of addiction, then it is safe to assume that the number of addicted caregivers, either active or in recovery, approximates 500,000. Thus, the question put to us focused on a clearly emerging trend in need of thoughtful exploration.

The burdens of caregiving mixed with the hardships of the caregiver's own recovery challenges often create "the perfect storm" of relapse. At first glance, it seems that relapse is inevitable for someone who must concentrate on their own sobriety to, quite literally, stay alive, yet is compelled to focus on the serious illness of a loved one instead. But in our view, the apparent bleakness of this situation is the result of a failure to recognize that the two worlds—the worlds of recovery and of caregiving—are meant to thrive together, not conflict with each other. They can also be hidden gifts for each other.

The disease of alcoholism is a three-headed monster. It is rooted in the biological, psychological and social worlds of those affected by it. The disease goes much further than being the monster of just the individual; this chronic and often terminal illness spreads its dark energy over the entire family system of the alcoholic: immediate, extended and even one's family of choice. It takes no prisoners. And unless the eye of the recovering alcoholic is always on the "sobriety ball," it is easy to slip into the gray world of relapse. Relapse does not begin with the alcoholic taking a drink, but instead by the alcoholic beginning to make the life-sacrificing choices that often serve as the first step toward that drink.

Caregiving seduces a recovering addict into taking his eye off the sobriety ball and instead fixes his attention on a loved one's world. That attention to another's needs is, in large measure, driven by need, guilt, shame or a combination of the three. Add to the challenging prognosis of any recovering alcoholic the burdens of caregiving and the distractions of the medical, social, financial and other needs of that family member or friend, and any chance of a successful recovery seems truly remote. Caregiving seems nearly impossible when following a plan to take care of oneself first. Recovery is nearly impossible when one is forced to spend one's life caring for another. When both are happening simultaneously, the results are often disastrous for everyone.

By definition, caregiving is a relationship in which one assumes the life tasks, schedules and activities of someone else. It can also be seen as the "set up beyond set ups" for a recovering person, because so many believe that to be a good caregiver one must care for another to the detriment of taking care of one's own mind, body and soul. In balancing the two, the recovering caregiver must solve the problem of knowing when to help and when not to help. A caregiver needs to know when to partner with the loved one and encourage him or her to meet the caregiver halfway.

Caregiving takes people out of their day-to-day communities, out of the flow of life. Caregivers often see themselves as martyrs, denying themselves everything in favor of the needs of the loved one, and in so doing take themselves out of the flow of their own healing. What could be worse for recovering alcoholics, who are being asked to immerse themselves in the A.A. community, work the steps with their sponsors and steadfastly attend meetings, than the inevitable isolation brought about by caregiving?

Yet, if caregivers can learn to take care of themselves, the act can be sacred and loving. It is about learning a new language, a new world and a new approach to life in general. Doesn't this sound so much like a person coming out of treatment, who must adhere to a new way of life as well? That is why we believe that a person who is strong in his or her own recovery efforts always makes the best caregiver.

Just as parents traveling with young children are instructed on airplane flights in case of emergency, at our foundation we tell caregivers to "take the oxygen first." It is the same advice we give to recovering clients: to "put their sobriety first." There really is no difference between the two and they are never in conflict, despite the selflessness that is thought to be required in caring for a loved one.

Recovery lasts a lifetime. It is akin to a marathon. Caregiving can last a few months or a few years, and is too often approached as if it were a sprint. Caregivers who do not take care of themselves mind, body and soul often die before the loved one they take care of. Recovering people have the greatest tools at their disposal to be able to finish the marathon successfully, rather than dying in the proverbial "sprint." "Sobriety first" is the recovering alcoholic's mantra and the caregiver's mantra is "take the oxygen first."

Without using the recovering community to immerse oneself in needed support, a recovering caregiver will have few answers to the questions of how to deal with the sadness, the change in family dynamics, the isolation, frustration, chaos, anxiety and depression that often accompany caregiving. I once overheard a sponsor telling his charge that his relapse was imminent because there was nothing in his "recovery bank" for him to draw on when life went awry. It is easy to stay sober when times are good, but a reserve of strength is vital when things go bad. The problems of caregiving will inevitably arise. Recovering caregivers know how to build that reserve. Using their community, their program and their sponsor are necessary to help build this reserve.

Powerful recovering caregivers are those who are strong in their own recovery. They have a plan, a program and a culture that is the antidote to isolation. They realize that to be a martyr is to begin entering the world of relapse. Those caregivers who use their programs of recovery as a guide to their caregiving experience see a sacred and heroic path instead of a depressing journey into a world of pain and martyrdom. Working a program of recovery ensures caregivers strength, fortitude and hope instead of pain. It also, as a byproduct, allows the carereciever to feel balanced and steady as he faces the challenges of daily living.

Thus the twelve-step program becomes the spring of hope recovering caregivers can always dive into. It is the power to make a difference. It is the spiritual way to solve a difficult problem. It is the knowledge that they have been tested by fire, and yet in the end, they know they will survive, because there is a plan to help them survive.

The program of recovery offers hope, gratitude and inspiration. It allows one to be honest, open and willing. It reduces guilt and shame. When alcoholics pay attention to their program of recovery while they provide ongoing care, they are more likely to recognize the value of what they are doing, even acknowledge and grow from the daily, individual achievements of tending to their loved one. Caregivers who stay close to their program of recovery gain a sense of self-confidence, a belief in their ability to have control over situations. The positive energy given off by the empowered caregiver allows the care receiver to feel safer and more balanced in his or her presence. The resulting security leads to a greater quality of care and a stronger family system.

Unfortunately, caregiving often becomes a part of our lives at a time when we have not developed an understanding of the underlying relationship issues we may already have with the loved one who now needs our care. The caregiver must be able to work with concepts such as forgiveness, letting go and boundaries. If you are not yet a caregiver, find a therapist to deal with those underlying family issues before the day arrives when you have to take care of that family member.

The assistance of a therapist and holding fast and true to a program of recovery is vital. Anything less is often just a half measure. It is your lifesaving strategy during a very challenging journey. Through this important combination, you will not only be able to save your own life but you also may become the beacon of hope for the family around you; saving others as a byproduct of your abundance.

It all begins with you. "Caregiver, heal thyself," and while you are at it, "take the oxygen first." If you are not sure where that oxygen is, find a community A.A. schedule and as soon as you finish this essay, go to a meeting! Find a therapist with whom you feel comfortable. Positive things usually unfold from there. Remember, a journey of a thousand miles begins with one step.

Dr. James Huysman is the co-founder and Executive Director of The Leeza Gibbons Memory Foundation, a non-profit organization dedicated to the education and empowerment of caregivers and their family members who suffer from long-term memory disorders. He is a psychologist, board certified therapist in clinical social work, crisis interventionist and nationally certified addictions professional. His varied career has included responsive advocacy, client care and progressive health services development. The recipient of a Psy.D. in psychology from the Southern California School of Professional Studies and a master's degree in social work from Barry University, he has developed national programs, and served as a clinical consultant and as an officer for a large number of national hospitals and independent psychiatric and addictions centers.

Send Us Your Story

Do you have a story to tell? LaChance Publishing and The Healing Project publish four books a year of stories written by people like you. Have you or those you know been touched by life-threatening illness or chronic disease? Your story can give comfort, courage and strength to others who are going through what you have already faced.

Your story should be no less than 500 words and no more than 2,000 words. You can write about yourself or someone you know. Your story must inform, inspire, or teach others. Tell the story of how you or someone you know faced adversity; what you learned that would be important for others to know; how dealing with the disease strengthened or clarified your relationships or inspired positive changes in your life.

The easiest way to submit your story is to visit the LaChance Publishing website at www.lachancepublishing.com. There you will find guidelines for submitting your story online, or you may write to us at submissions@lachancepublishing.com. We look forward to reading your story!

Resources

On the following pages you will find information on some of the foremost organizations in the country focused on alcoholism research, treatment and support. All of these and many, many more may be found within the Resources Section of The Healing Project's website at www.thehealingproject.org.

National Organizations for Substance Abuse and Addiction

American Council on Alcoholism (ACA)
1000 E. Indian School Road
Phoenix, AZ 85014
Toll Free Number: 1-800-527-5344
Fax: (602) 264-7403
Email: info@aca-usa.org
http://www.aca-usa.org/alcoholism.htm

An information and referral service for individuals who suffer from alcohol dependence, their families, treatment professionals and the general public who are seeking a broad range of information on alcohol, alcohol dependence, alcohol abuse and options for recovery.

The National Center on Addiction and Substance Abuse (CASA)
633 Third Avenue, 19th Floor
New York, NY 10017-6706
Phone: (212) 841-5200

http://www.casacolumbia.org

The only nationwide organization that brings together under one roof all of the professional disciplines needed to study and combat the abuse of all substances—alcohol and nicotine as well as illegal, prescription and performance enhancing drugs—in all sectors of society.

Mayo Clinic:
Jacksonville, Florida
4500 San Pablo Road
Jacksonville, FL 32224
General Number: (904) 953-2000
Hearing Impaired (TDD): (904) 953-2300
Appointment Office: (904) 953-0853/Fax (904) 953-2898
International Services: (904) 953-7329

St. Luke's Hospital
4201 Belfort Road
Jacksonville, FL 32222
General Number: (904) 296-3700

Rochester, Minnesota
Mayo Clinic
200 First Street S.W.
Rochester, MN 55905
General Number: (507) 284-2511
Fax: (507) 284-0161
Hearing Impaired: (507) 284-9786
Appointment Office: (507) 538-3270
International Services: (507) 284-8884/Fax: (507) 284-3891

Rochester Methodist Hospital
201 West Center Street
Rochester, MN 55902
General Number: (507) 266-7890

Saint Mary's Hospital including Mayo
 Eugenio Litta Children's Hospital
1222 Second Street S.W.
Rochester, MN 55902
General Number: (507) 255-5123

Scottsdale/Phoenix, Arizona
Mayo Clinic
13400 East Shea Boulevard
Scottsdale, AZ 85259
General Number: (480) 301-8000
Fax: (480) 301-7006
Appointment Office: 1-800-446-2279
International Patients Center: (480) 301-7101
Fax: (480) 301-9310

Mayo Clinic Hospital
5777 East Mayo Boulevard
Phoenix, AZ 85054
General Number: (480) 515-6296
Hearing Impaired: (480) 342-0169
Business Office Fax: (480) 342-1138

A not-for-profit medical practice dedicated to the diagnosis and treatment of virtually every type of complex illness. Mayo Clinic staff members work together to meet your needs. You will see as many doctors, specialists and other health care professionals as needed to provide a comprehensive diagnosis, understandable answers and effective treatment.

National Association of Addiction Treatment Providers
313 W. Liberty Street, Suite 129
Lancaster, PA 17603-2748
Phone: (717) 392-8480
Fax: (717) 392-8481
Email: rhunsicker@naatp.org

http://www.naatp.org

Provides ethical, research-based treatment for alcoholism and other drug addictions and provides its members and the public with accurate, responsible information and other resources related to the treatment of addiction.

National Council on Alcoholism and Drug Dependence, Inc.
244 East 58th Street, 4th Floor
New York, NY 10022
Phone: (212) 269-7797
Fax: (212) 269-7510
Email: national@ncadd.org
HOPE LINE: 1-800/NCA-CALL (24-hour Affiliate referral)
http://www.ncadd.org

NCADD provides education, information, help and hope to the public through its advocacy of prevention, intervention and treatment through a nationwide network of affiliate organizations.

National Institute on Alcohol Abuse and Alcoholism
5635 Fishers Lane, MSC 9304
Bethesda, MD 20892-9304
Communications/Public Info: (301) 443-3860
Toll Free Number: 1-800-662-HELP ENG/ESP
Email: niaaaweb-r@exchange.nih.gov
http://www.niaaa.nih.gov/Resources/RelatedWebsites/
   Referral.htm

NIAAA provides leadership in the national effort to reduce alcohol-related problems by conducting and supporting research in a wide range of scientific areas including genetics, neuroscience, epidemiology, prevention and treatment. It coordinates and collaborates with other research institutes and federal programs on alcohol-related issues and with international, national, state and local institutions, organizations, agencies and programs engaged in alcohol-related work translating and disseminating research findings to health care providers, researchers, policymakers and the public.

Information on Alcoholism

National Clearinghouse for Alcohol and Drug Information
P.O. Box 2345
Rockville, MD 20847-2345
Toll Free Number: 1-800-729-6686 (English and Español)
Hearing Impaired: 1-800-487-4889 (TDD)
http://www.ncadi.samsha.gov

Provides information about substance abuse, prevention and treatment. It employs both English and Spanish-speaking information specialists skilled at recommending appropriate publications, posters and videocassettes, conducting customized searches, providing grant and funding information and referring people to appropriate organizations.

American Council on Alcoholism (ACA)
1000 E. Indian School Road
Phoenix, AZ 85014
Toll Free Number: 1-800-527-5344
Fax: (602) 264-7403
Email: info@aca-usa.org
http://www.aca-usa.org/alcoholism.htm

National Council on Alcoholism and Drug Dependence, Inc.
244 East 58th Street, 4th Floor
New York, NY 10022
Phone: (212) 269-7797
Fax: (212) 269-7510
Email: national@ncadd.org
HOPE LINE: 1-800-NCA-CALL (24-hour Affiliate referral)
http://www.ncadd.org

Legal Help

Legal Action Center, Washington D.C. Office
236 Massachusetts Avenue NE, Suite 505
Washington, D.C. 20002-4980
Phone: (202) 544-5478
Fax: (202) 544-5712
Email: lacdc@lac-dc.org
http://www.lac.org

The only non-profit law and policy organization in the United States whose sole mission is to fight discrimination against people with histories of addiction, HIV/AIDS or criminal records, and to advocate for sound public policies in these areas.

U.S. Department of Health and Human Services
200 Independence Avenue, S.W.
Washington, D.C. 20201
Toll Free Number: 1-800-729-6686
Hearing Impaired (TDD): 1-800-487-4889
Español: 1-877-767-8432
https://ncadistore.samhsa.gov/catalog/productDetails.aspx?ProductID=16968

Its publications help those in recovery understand their rights under Federal laws protecting against discrimination, including information about the legal consequences of alcohol and drug-related conduct that can limit rights and opportunities and what an individual can do to prevent or remedy violations and overcome barriers due to past or current drug- or alcohol-related conduct.

Support Groups

A.A. World Services, Inc.
P.O. Box 459
New York, NY 10163
Phone: (212) 870-3400

http://www.alcoholics-anonymous.org/

Alcoholics Anonymous is a fellowship of men and women who share their experience, strength and hope with each other so that they may solve their common problems and help others to recover from alcoholism. The only requirement for membership is a desire to stop drinking. A.A. is not allied with any sect, denomination, politics, organization or institution; it does not wish to engage in any controversy; and neither endorses nor opposes any causes. Its primary purpose is to help alcoholics to achieve sobriety.

National Clearinghouse for Alcohol and Drug Information (NCADI)
P.O. Box 2345
Rockville, MD 20847-2345
Toll Free Number: 1-800-729-6686 (English and Spanish)
Hearing Impaired: 1-800-487-4889 (TDD)
http://www.ncadi.samsha.gov

SMART Recovery® Central Office
7537 Mentor Avenue, Suite #306
Mentor, OH 44060
Phone: (440) 951-5357
Toll Free Number: (866) 951-5357
Fax: (440) 951-5358
Email: info@smartrecovery.org
http://www.smartrecovery.org

Offers support for individuals who have chosen to abstain, or are considering abstinence, from any type of addictive behaviors (substances or activities), by teaching how to change self-defeating thinking, emotions and actions and to work towards long-term satisfactions and quality of life.

Residential Treatment Centers

Caron Treatment Centers
P.O. Box 150
Wernersville, PA 19565
Toll Free Number: 1-800-678-2332
http://www.caron.org/

A not-for-profit organization the mission of which is to provide an enlightened and caring treatment community in which all those affected by alcoholism or other drug addiction may begin a new life.

Hazelden Foundation
CO3, P.O. Box 11
Center City, MN 55012-0011
Phone: 1-800-257-7810 or (651) 213-4200
Fax: (651) 213-4411
Email: info@hazelden.org
http://www.hazelden.org

For individuals, families and communities struggling with addiction to alcohol and other drugs. Thousands of people from all 50 states and 42 foreign countries have turned to Hazelden to find expertise, quality care and the leading authorities on addiction and recovery issues.

The Salvation Army National Headquarters
615 Slaters Lane
P.O. Box 269
Alexandria, VA 22313
Email: NHQ_Webmaster@usn.salvationarmy.org
http://www.satruck.org/FindARC.aspx

For over 100 years The Salvation Army has been providing assistance to people with a variety of social and spiritual afflictions through its 119 United States-based adult rehabilitation centers.

The Scripps Research Institute Alcohol Research Center
10550 North Torrey Pines Road, SR 401A
La Jolla, CA 92037
Phone: (858) 784-1000
Email: arcadmin@scripps.edu
http://arc.scripps.edu

Scripps is committed to improving the understanding of the biological and psychological causes of alcoholism and aims to answer the questions of what alcoholism is and why alcoholism tends to be an ongoing issue in people's lives.

Triangle Residential Options for Substance Abusers, Inc. (TROSA)
1820 James Street
Durham, NC 27707
Phone: (919) 419-1059
http://www.trosainc.org

A comprehensive, long-term, residential substance abuse recovery program that includes vocational training, education, communication, peer counseling, mentoring, leadership training and aftercare. The program is provided at no cost to the individual.

Volunteers of America
1660 Duke Street
Alexandria, VA 22314
Toll Free Number: 1-800-899-0089
Phone: (703) 341-5000
Fax: (703) 341-7000
http://www.voa.org/ourservices/substanceabuse

Volunteers of America offers a continuum of support services and residential treatment options to assist adolescents, adults and their families to experience life without addiction and become contributing members of their communities.

Women's Organizations

Mercy Ministries
Mercy Ministries of America
Corporate Office
P.O. Box 111060
Nashville, TN 37222-1060
Phone: (615) 831-6987
Fax: (615) 315-9749
Email: info@mercyministries.com
http://www.mercyministries.org

A residential program for young women between the ages of 13 and 28 dealing with life-controlling issues.

New Directions for Women
2607 Willo Avenue
Costa Mesa, CA 92627
Toll Free Number: 1-800-93-WOMEN or 1-800-939-6636
Email: contact@newdirectionsforwomen.org
http://www.newdirectionsforwomen.org

A drug and alcohol treatment provider offering services for women, pregnant women, and women with children.

Organizations for Youth and Children

Al-Anon/Alateen
1600 Corporate Landing Parkway
Virginia Beach, VA 23454-5617
Phone: (757) 563-1600
Fax: (757) 563-1655

Al-Anon offers hope and help to the families and friends of alcoholics.

The Betty Ford Center
39000 Bob Hope Drive
Rancho Mirage, CA 92270
Phone: (760) 773-4100
Toll Free Number: 1-800-434-7365
http://www.bettyfordcenter.org/children/

The Betty Ford Center children's program helps children ages 7 to 12 from families suffering from addiction. No child is turned away for lack of funds. Scholarships are available. Parents do not have to be patients at the Betty Ford Center in order for their children to participate in the program.

Caron
P.O. Box 150
Wernersville, PA 19565
Toll Free Number: 1-800-678-2332
http://www.caron.org/header.asp?section=adolescent&cat=ps-adolescent

Its Adolescent Programs provide accurate drug and alcohol assessment and address co-occurring psychiatric issues while simultaneously meeting increasingly complicated family needs.

Jeffrey S. Wolfsberg & Associates, Inc.
Canton, MA 02021
Phone: (508) 728-1706
Email: contact@jeffwolfsberg.com
http://www.jeffwolfsberg.com/new_pages/contactus.html

A privately owned consulting firm that works with independent schools (K-12) worldwide to design, implement and sustain effective prevention strategies for the reduction of underage drinking, drug use, and bullying among children and adolescents.

Free or Low-Cost Treatment

The Betty Ford Center
39000 Bob Hope Drive
Rancho Mirage, CA 92270
Phone: (760) 773-4100
Toll Free Number: 1-800-434-7365
http://www.bettyfordcenter.org

Triangle Residential Options for Substance Abusers, Inc.
1820 James Street
Durham, NC 27707
Phone: (919) 419-1059
http://www.trosainc.org

Recovery Schools

Association of Recovery Schools
P.O. Box 128576
Nashville, TN 37212
Phone: (615) 812-0379
http://www.recoveryschools.org

Advocates for the promotion, strengthening and expansion of secondary and post-secondary programs designed for students and families committed to achieving success in both education and recovery.

For the duration of the printing and circulation of this book, for every book that is sold by LaChance Publishing, LaChance will contribute 100% of the net proceeds to The Healing Project, LLC. The Healing Project can be reached at Five Laurel Road, South Salem, NY 10590. The Healing Project is dedicated to promoting the health and well-being of individuals suffering from life-threatening illnesses and chronic diseases, developing resources to enhance their quality of life and assisting the family members and friends who care for them. The Healing Project is a tax exempt organization as defined in Internal Revenue Code Section 501(c)(3).